BIOPHARMACEUTICALS

Edited by **Ming-Kung Yeh**
and **Yuan-Chuan Chen**

Biopharmaceuticals
http://dx.doi.org/10.5772/intechopen.72960
Edited by Ming-Kung Yeh and Yuan-Chuan Chen

Contributors

Alberto Pais, Carla Vitorino, Jéssica Silva, Ana Miranda, João Sousa, Jung-Keun Suh, Woojeong Kim, Kui Hyun Kang, Cedric Schirmer, Thomas Nussbaumer, Reto Schöb, Ralf Pörtner, Dieter Eibl, Regine Eibl, Po-Chih Wu, Der-Yuan Wang, Hwei-Fang Cheng, Yi-Chen Yang, Pavel Makarevich, Georgy Sagaradze, Anastasia Efimenko, Zhanna Akopyan, Pyotr Nimiritsky, Ming-Kung Yeh, Yuan-Chuan Chen

First published in London, United Kingdom, 2018 by IntechOpen
IntechOpen is the global imprint of INTECHOPEN LIMITED, registered in England and Wales, registration number: 11086078, The Shard, 25th floor, 32 London Bridge Street
London, SE19SG – United Kingdom
Printed in Croatia

British Library Cataloguing-in-Publication Data
A catalogue record for this book is available from the British Library

Additional hard copies can be obtained from orders@intechopen.com

Biopharmaceuticals, Edited by Ming-Kung Yeh and Yuan-Chuan Chen
p. cm.
Print ISBN 978-1-78923-718-4
Online ISBN 978-1-78923-719-1

For EU product safety concerns:
IN TECH d.o.o., Prolaz Marije Krucifikse Kozulić 3, 51000 Rijeka, Croatia,
info@intechopen.com or visit our website at intechopen.com.

Meet the editors

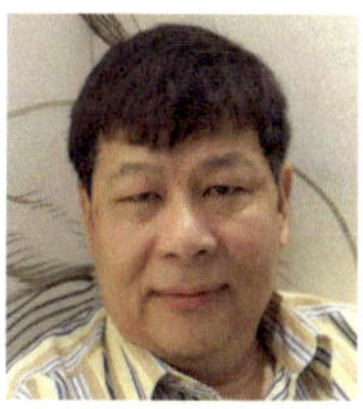

Ming-Kung Yeh gained his Bachelor and Master degrees from the National Defense Medical Center, Taiwan in 1986 and 1988, respectively. He completed his PhD at the University of Nottingham, UK, in 1996. From 1988 to 2008, he worked in the Tri-Service General Hospital, Taiwan from a basic pharmacist to a chief pharmacist and became a Professor of Preventive Medicine in 2008. He was the Head of the Pharmaceutical Administration, Ministry of National Defense, Taiwan, from 2011 to 2013. He was the General Director of the Taiwan Food and Drug Administration (TFDA), Ministry of Health and Welfare (MOHW) from 2013 to 2014, and a superintendent in MOHW from 2014 to 2016. His research focuses on public food and drug safety, and he also takes an active interest in pharmacy education, practice, and policy. Currently, he is devoting himself to developing cell therapy products.

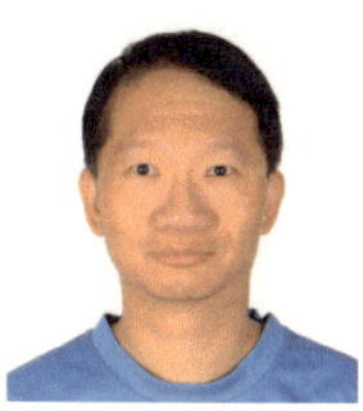

Yuan-Chuan Chen completed his PhD in Biochemistry at the University of California, Berkeley, USA, in 2015 and had postdoctoral studies at the Taiwan Food and Drug Administration (TFDA) from 2015 to 2016. His research interests include pharmacy, biochemistry, microbiology/virology, cell/molecule biology, biotechnology/nanotechnology, cell /gene therapy, and policy/regulation. His studies focus on the discovery, production, application, perspectives, and challenges of biopharmaceuticals. Additionally, he is interested in basic research, the development of agricultural/industrial products, and human therapeutics using the CRISPR/Cas9 system.

Contents

Preface

Health is priceless and to be free from illness is considered a basic human right. Along with the advance of biomedical science and the improvement of public health, many previously incorrigible diseases can be cured or even eradicated now and the life expectancy is definitely extended. Translational medicine linking the basic research and clinical applications promotes the discovery of novel medicines, particularly biopharmaceuticals. Clearly, biopharmaceuticals play an important role in the exciting development and progress of medicines. For recent studies, innovative biopharmaceuticals are developing rapidly and have opened a new era for human therapy. Many researchers are involved in the related research for the development of biopharmaceuticals and have achieved significant results. Our team has also been working on the same topics for years and has achieved some promising results. We have long hoped to summarize the research achievement of biopharmaceuticals in a book. Here, we are grateful for IntechOpen's generosity and enthusiasm to offer this opportunity to us.

Biopharmaceuticals, which consist of sugars, proteins, nucleic acids, living cells, or tissues, are medicinal products manufactured from extracted or semisynthesized biological sources like humans, animals, or microorganisms. Biopharmaceuticals have been extensively used as therapeutic agents such as vaccines, whole blood (or blood components), immunosera, antigens, hormones, cytokines, enzymes, allergenics, cell therapies, gene therapies, tissues, monoclonal antibodies, products derived from recombinant DNA, etc. For example, vaccines are used to prevent infectious diseases and some cancers; gene-based and cellular biopharmaceuticals are applied to treat a variety of diseases for which no other drugs or medical devices are available. However, the research and development (R&D) of biopharmaceuticals is typically difficult, expensive, and time-consuming. Biopharmaceuticals can be produced in microbial cells, animal cell lines, plant cell cultures, or bioreactors of various configurations. The cost of production (low-volume containers and high-purity products are essential) and microbial contamination are the two major concerns during the production process. Despite this, more and more biopharmaceuticals have been successfully developed and marketed through the introduction of new biotechnologies, production approaches, and delivery tools. The inventors who discover a new biopharmaceutical usually apply for a patent (or license) to have the grant for the exclusive manufacturing right, because this is a method by which the inventors can recover their investment cost. It is crucial to establish a strict but flexible framework of regulation for investigating, applying, and patenting biopharmaceuticals. Therefore, the interdisciplinary collaboration including researchers, regulators, funders, and manufacturers should be encouraged for the successful development of biopharmaceuticals.

Finally, we acknowledge the authors' participation in helping us to complete this book. Many professionals contributed their efforts, knowledge, and experiences to this publication. This book provides a platform to promote the sharing of experiences, the international cooperation and harmonization, and the presentation of research achievement. The readers will be able to read many constructive, insightful, and significant articles in the book. We wish that the researchers' accomplishments can be put into practice and improve the health of people worldwide in the future.

Ming-Kung Yeh, PhD
School of Pharmacy
National Defense Medical Center
Taipei, Taiwan

Yuan-Chuan Chen, PhD
Program in Comparative Biochemistry
University of California
Berkeley, CA, USA

Section 1

Background

Chapter 1

Introductory Chapter: Biopharmaceuticals

Yuan-Chuan Chen and Ming-Kung Yeh

Additional information is available at the end of the chapter

http://dx.doi.org/10.5772/intechopen.79194

1. Introduction

A biopharmaceutical (biological or biologic), which consists of sugars, proteins, nucleic acids, living cells, or tissues, is a medicinal product manufactured in extracted or semi-synthesized from biological sources like humans, animals, or microorganisms. Different from traditional drugs synthesized from chemical processes, the majority of biopharmaceutical products are derived from biological processes including the extraction from living systems or the production by recombinant DNA technologies (**Table 1**). Transgenic organisms, especially plants, animals, or microorganisms that have been genetically modified, are potentially used to produce biopharmaceuticals.

The recombinant human insulin (trade name "Humulin") was the first biopharmaceutical approved for human therapeutic uses and marketing in 1982. Currently, biopharmaceuticals have been extensively used as therapeutic agents such as vaccines, whole blood (or blood components), immunosera, antigens, hormones, cytokines, enzymes, allergenics, cell therapies, gene therapies, tissues, monoclonal antibodies, and products derived from recombinant DNA, etc. For example, vaccines are used to prevent infectious diseases and some cancers; cell- and gene-based biopharmaceuticals are applied to treat a variety of diseases for which no other drugs or medical devices are available.

The European Medicines Agency (EMA) uses the specific term "advanced therapy medicinal products (ATMPs)" to refer to human medicines that are based on cells, genes, or tissue engineering. Cell therapy products (CTPs) are biomedicines containing cells/tissues that have been manipulated to change their biological characteristics, and these cells/tissues can be used to treat, prevent, or diagnose diseases [1]. Gene therapy products (GTPs) are therapeutic agents to make genetic improvement through the repair, deletion, insertion, or substitution of mutated genes or site-specific modifications for target therapies [2]. Tissue engineering is the application of a combination of cell, engineering, and material methods, and suitable factors

Source item	Extracted from living systems	Produced by recombinant DNA
Characteristic	1. Some conventional biopharmaceuticals are extracted from animals or humans particularly. 2. Some biopharmaceuticals were extracted from animals, but they are currently produced by biotechnologies. For example, the therapeutic insulin previously extracted from porcine pancreatic islets is now produced by recombinant DNA technologies in the yeast (*Saccharomyces cerevisiae*) or *E. coli*.	Biopharmaceuticals produced by recombinant DNA technologies are usually one of the following three types: 1. Substances that are almost identical to the body's own key signaling proteins. 2. Monoclonal antibodies that are similar to the antibodies produced by the human immune system against microbes. 3. Receptor constructs (fusion proteins) that are usually based on a naturally occurring receptor linked to the immunoglobulin frame.
Example	Whole blood and blood components, organs and tissue transplants, stem cells, antibodies for passive immunization, fecal microbiota, human breast milk, human reproductive cells	Blood factors, tissue plasminogen activators, hormones, hematopoietic growth factors, interferons, interleukin-based products, vaccines, monoclonal antibodies, tumor necrosis factors, therapeutic enzymes

Table 1. Major sources of biopharmaceuticals.

are added to improve, repair, or replace only part of or whole biological tissues such as bones, cartilages, blood vessels, organs, skins, muscles, etc. It also involves the use of a tissue scaffold for the formation of new viable tissues for medical purposes [3–5].

A biosimilar, also known as "follow-on biologic," is a biologic medical product that is almost identical to a copy of an original product manufactured by different pharmaceutical companies. It is highly similar to a licensed reference product in spite of minor differences in clinically inactive components. There are no clinically significant differences between the biosimilars and the reference products in terms of the safety, purity, and potency. A generic drug is the same as a brand name drug in dosage, safety, strength, administration, quality, performance, and intended uses. It is required to take a lot of rigorous tests to ensure that the generic drug can substitute for the brand name drug. A generic drug must contain identical active pharmaceutical ingredients (APIs) with the same amount as the brand name product and be proved to be bioequivalent to the brand name drug. The substitutability or therapeutic equivalence of generic drugs has to be evaluated scientifically. If a generic drug is evaluated as therapeutically equivalent as the brand name product, it has equal effects and show no differences compared with the brand name product. Biosimilars, like generic drugs, can be manufactured when the original "innovator" product's patent expires, and are officially approved versions of the original products [6]. However, there are many differences between a generic drug and a biosimilar (**Table 2**). Biosimilars have the same clinical effect as generic drugs but are only similar to the original "innovator" drugs as they are confirmed by validation methods. Biosimilars will not be the same as the reference products, unlike generic drugs in which the APIs are identical to the references [7]. Despite this heterogeneity, all generic drugs and biosimilars have to maintain consistent quality and effective performance throughout their life cycles [8].

Drug property	Generic drug	Biosimilar
Molecular size	Small (~150 Da)	Large (~150,000 Da)
Structure	Simple and well-defined	Complex with probable structural variations
Characterization	Easy	Difficult
Stability	More stable for storage and handling	Less stable, very sensitive to its surroundings
Production	Predictable chemical processes are used to manufacture an identical copy	Specialized biological processes are used to manufacture a similar copy
Identical to reference products	Yes	No
	At least, active pharmaceutical ingredients are identical	Minor differences in clinically inactive components are acceptable
Adverse immune responses	Lower potential	Higher potential
Frequency of quality tests in manufacturing	≤50	≥250
Clinical trials requirement for approval	Small clinical trials in healthy volunteers	Large clinical trials in patients
Discovery cost	Low or even no	Relatively high

Table 2. Comparison of a generic drug and a biosimilar.

2. Application

Biopharmaceuticals have multiple clinical applications and various advantages for disease therapy, prevention, and diagnosis.

2.1. Therapy

The therapeutic types of biopharmaceuticals mainly include recombinant protein therapy, antibody therapy, cell therapy, and gene therapy. Biopharmaceuticals are able to cure or treat diseases safely and effectively by demonstrating biological activity, and perform specific functions by acting on the disease pathophysiology. Compared with chemical drugs, biopharmaceuticals are more complex in production, have multiple routes of administration and different pharmacokinetics. Their advantages are high selectivity and low nonspecific toxicity; disadvantages include high costs and the induction of antidrug antibodies leading to decreased efficacy or deficiency in biosafety. Treatment can be optimized through the development of dosing schedules and multiple administrative routes. Additionally, the cost can be reduced by using biosimilars.

2.2. Prevention

A vaccine is the most important biopharmaceutical used for infectious disease prevention. It usually contains a biological agent that resembles a pathogen and is usually made from inactivated microbes, live attenuated microbes, toxoids (toxins), and or part of surface antigens (subunits). Through vaccination, the burst of many infectious diseases has enormously been decreased such as measles, tetanus, and polio; some are even eradicated such as smallpox. However, the burden of noninfectious diseases such as cancers, cardiovascular diseases, metabolic diseases, and neurodegenerative diseases is significantly increasing. Currently, some vaccines are successfully applied to prevent cancers; for example, the human papilloma virus (HPV) vaccine has been approved for the prevention of cervical cancers.

2.3. Diagnosis

In addition to clinic significance in therapy and prevention, some biopharmaceuticals can be used to diagnose diseases; for example, monoclonal antibodies have been successfully applied in the diagnosis of some cancers and infectious diseases, and more are being developed [9–11]. Once monoclonal antibodies specified for a given substance are produced, they can be used to detect the presence of this substance. They are also very useful in immunohistochemistry that detects antigens in fixed tissue sections and immunofluorescence tests that detect the substance in frozen tissue sections or in live cells.

3. Perspective and challenge

For recent studies, innovative biopharmaceuticals are developing rapidly and have opened a new era for human therapy. Many researchers involve in the development of biopharmaceuticals and achieve exciting results. Biopharmaceuticals are promising for scientific perspectives and regulatory perspectives. Nonetheless, there are still some challenges including scientific issues and regulatory issues we need to overcome.

3.1. Scientific issue

Along with the advance of biotechnologies, more novel biopharmaceuticals are marketed and used for clinical application in the world. Biopharmaceuticals have been extensively applied for disease control, prevention, and diagnosis even though some scientific challenges are still unsolved. Take vaccines and gene therapies as examples to discuss as follows:

3.1.1. Vaccine

Vaccination, the administration of an antigenic material (vaccine), is considered to be the most effective strategies for disease control. Appropriate formulation and delivery of vaccines can maximize the potential advances for disease prevention. The main advantages of vaccination include the prevention in advance and the immunity for long term; the limitations are complex vaccination schedules, strict requirements for storage, and restricted routes of administration [12]. Nanotechnology is an approach to prepare a nanovaccine with the consumption and side effects significantly decreased. Through the application of nanoparticles, it is possible for vaccines to be controlled release at specific location, stable at room temperature, and have replaceable routes for administration. Vaccines based on nanotechnologies may overcome their limitations and result in the development of painless, safe, effective, and economic products. The major challenges are the toxicity of nanoparticles and the immune responses induced by nanoparticles, though some biodegradable and biocompatible nanoparticles have been developed [12].

Biotechnologies using recombinant DNA technologies, genetic engineering, and tissue culture encompass a wide range of procedures to modify living organisms for human uses. New vaccines employing biotechnologies improve the product quality and expand the clinical applications [13]. For example, traditional vaccines are only used to prevent infectious diseases, but vaccines based on biotechnologies are being developed to prevent many noninfectious diseases such as cancers, type I diabetes mellitus (T1DM), Alzheimer disease, drug addiction, etc. [13]. In addition, therapeutic vaccines are potentially developing for both infectious and noninfectious diseases using the biotechnologies such as reverse vaccinology, recombinant subunit vaccination, recombinant protein vaccination, DNA vaccination, and RNA vaccination. The major challenge is complex vaccination schedules. The vaccines based on biotechnologies are usually only parts of microorganisms (DNA, RNA, or protein); therefore, it is required to have multiple doses to induce additional "booster" shots for full immunity [13].

3.1.2. *Gene therapy*

Although many CTPs have been approved for marketing in many countries and extensively used for disease treatment [1], current gene therapies predominantly exist in basic research laboratories and their clinical applications are still on trials. Despite of this, some GTPs have been approved by the EMA such as Glybera (alipogene tiparvovec) in 2012, and by the United States Food and Drug Administration (US FDA) such as Kymriah (tisagenlecleucel) and Yescarta (axicabtagene ciloleucel) in 2017, respectively. Recently, gene therapies have become possible through the advances of genetic engineering technology that enabled the manipulation of genome and the development of delivery tools such as lipoids [2, 14], viruses [2, 14], nanoparticles [2, 14], bacteria [15], gene guns [16], electroporation [17], or nanostraws [18]. Therapeutic components must be transported to targeted cells to exert a therapeutic effect. Therefore, the delivery tool is essential for drug delivery to target cells and it is very crucial to select a suitable delivery tool with specificity, efficiency, safety, and economics. However, it is challenging for the option of delivery tools due to the following issues.

1. Specificity: Some delivery tools are not very specific and may deliver nucleic acids to non-target cells. It is important to reduce the risk of nonspecific delivery, but the evaluation of their benefits and risks is complex.

2. Efficiency: Not all delivery tools are efficient enough; some of them are low in efficiency and multiple rounds of transfections are needed. Additionally, it is hard to improve and evaluate their efficiency especially in animals and clinics.

3. Biosafety: Some delivery tools are toxic, biohazardous, or even destructive to normal cells or recipient hosts. Some delivery tools such as lipoids, viruses, bacteria, and nanoparticles may induce vector-associated immune responses in hosts, and to overcome immune barriers is essential [14]. Consequently, it is required to verify their safety in preliminary tests.

4. Economics: The research and development (R&D) of delivery tools is perhaps difficult, risky, costly, and time-consuming. Consequently, researchers, funders, and manufacturers must have enough incentives to develop delivery tools. In fact, most biotechnology companies have little incentive to discover novel delivery tools because of limited revenue and highly developmental risks.

In several recent studies, encouraging progresses have been made to possibly overcome the challenges of delivering GTPs *in vivo* [19–22] (**Table 3**).

3.2. Regulatory issue

Biopharmaceuticals are more complex than small molecular-weight drugs due to their biological source, large molecular size, structural complexity, and environmental sensitivity. Thus, it is essential to consider specific and special regulatory issues for the research, production, clinical trials, applications, and marketing of biopharmaceuticals, though many professional regulations and developmental frameworks have already been established. Take cell therapies and gene therapies, and biosimilars as examples to discuss as follows:

3.2.1. Cell therapy and gene therapy

CTPs and GTPs have the trend to be commodified because many manufacturers are aiming at pursuing commercial interests. Commercial promotion of unsupported therapeutic uses of CTPs and GTPs has become global challenges that have proven resistant to regulatory efforts. Some unapproved or unproved CTPs and GTPs are tried on patients only according to their indefinite perspectives. Some CTPs and GTPs which clinical trials or data are still incomplete are prematurely released on the market only due to significant interests. A coordinated approach at the national and international levels focused on engagement, harmonization, and enforcement must be implemented to reduce the risks related to direct consumer marketing of unapproved or unproven CTPs and GTPs [23]. However, in some cases, some CTPs or GTPs have not yet completed their efficacy validation, but they have enough data to verify their

Challenge	Strategy
Specificity	Discovery of a specific virus such as adeno-associated viruses (AAVs)
Efficiency	Application of a combination system such as AAVs-CRISPRs
Biosafety	Combination with several factors such as smaller Cas9 orthologues, tissue-specific minimal promoters, AAV serotypes, and different routes of administration;
	Development of novel and safe delivery tools such as lipid nanoparticles (LNPs), AAVs, and baculoviruses
Economics	International collaboration among manufacturers and harmonization for product review and approval in different countries can raise the profits and reduce the expenses

Abbreviation: clustered regularly interspaced short palindromic repeats (CRISPRs)/Cas9 nuclease system.

Table 3. Possible strategies for overcoming the challenges for drug delivery (cited from **Table 3**. Potential Application of the CRISPR/Cas9 System against Herpesvirus Infections. Viruses. 2018 May 29;**10**(6). pii: E291).

safety and estimate their efficacy. For the therapy of patents, who are in serious conditions or unmet medical needs, specific CTPs or GTPs can be accessible to these patients with adaptive licensing [1]. The regulator should establish a conditional approval system in the regulation with deadline, a fast-track review, and communication mechanism to have patients in urgent needs take specific CTPs or GTPs as soon as possible.

3.2.2. *Biosimilar*

As products of living organisms, biopharmaceuticals are more complicated than small molecular-weight chemical drugs because of their sensitivity to manufacturing processes and post-translational changes [24]. Most information on the manufacturing process is not fully open to the public, because it may be proprietary or a patent. This information gap stands for a critical challenge for biosimilar developers and plays a crucial role in explaining the differences in regulatory pathways. It is required to demonstrate biosimilarity and assure that the change in manufacturing process represents no effects on safety and efficacy. The extent of the change is usually a key indicator to the analysis required to evaluate the quality. Biosimilarity exercises have been addressed differently by regulators to realize that biosimilar developers begin with fundamental differences including culture media, purification processes, and formulations [24]. Therefore, it is required to ensure that the changes do not influence the efficacy and safety of biosimilars.

Biosimilars are defined and present their financial and clinical implications in current publications, regulations, and the US FDA guidance documents [25]. Some biopharmaceuticals may be replaced with cheaper biosimilars when they lose the patent protection. However, unlike generic drugs, biosimilars are different from the reference products in structure and function. The US Biologics Price Competition and Innovation (BPCI) Act of 2009 created an abbreviated licensure pathway to allow for the development and approval of biosimilars and interchangeable reference products that are licensed [25, 26]. The US FDA can approve biosimilars via the abbreviated licensure pathway in accordance with the BPCI Act. Biosimilars approved in Europe are only composed of simple and small molecules. Complex and large-molecule biosimilars will be subjected to a more rigorous and prolonged approval processes [25]. The financial success of biopharmaceutical therapies and their patent expiration eventually result in the development of biosimilars. The pharmaceutical company has to develop complex biosimilars that mimic the original "innovator" drugs and explore analytical methods to demonstrate similarity to regulatory authorities [25]. A comment outlines the efforts of an integrated health system to ensure biosimilar accessibility and discusses the current challenges and future implications [27]. Biosimilars still confront regulatory challenges on potential implications for pricing, site of care, and pharmacy dispensing practices [27]. Generally, we believe that biosimilars are helpful to the health-care system, but their expected benefits may not be understood in the near future.

4. Conclusion

Biopharmaceuticals are very promising for disease control and prevention due to their characteristics and multiple advantages over traditional drugs. Many novel biopharmaceuticals are being developed and may be applied for clinical application in the near future, though some scientific and regulatory issues are still unsolved. We expect research works including the discovery, production, applications, prospects, and challenges of biopharmaceuticals to gain the fruitful outcome and have a great impact over the humans. All prospects will come true and challenges will be overcome eventually if we constantly endeavor.

Author details

Yuan-Chuan Chen[1,2] and Ming-Kung Yeh[3]*

*Address all correspondence to: mkyeh2004@gmail.com

1 Program in Comparative Biochemistry, University of California, Berkeley, CA, USA

2 National Applied Research Laboratories, Taipei, Taiwan

3 School of Pharmacy, National Defense Medical Center, Taipei, Taiwan

References

[1] Chen YC, Cheng HF, Yeh MK. Cell therapy regulation in Taiwan. Cell Transplantation. 2017;**26**(3):483-492. DOI: 10.3727/096368916X693293

[2] Gonçalves GAR, Paiva RMA. Gene therapy: Advances, challenges and perspectives. Einstein (Sao Paulo). 2017;**15**(3):369-375. DOI: 10.1590/S1679-45082017RB4024

[3] Marei MK, El Backly RM. Dental mesenchymal stem cell-based translational regenerative dentistry: From artificial to biological replacement. Frontiers in Bioengineering and Biotechnology. 2018;**6**:49. DOI: 10.3389/fbioe.2018.00049

[4] Shoji T, Shinoka T. Tissue engineered vascular grafts for pediatric cardiac surgery. Translational Pediatrics. 2018;**7**(2):188-195. DOI: 10.21037/tp.2018.02.01

[5] Stephenson M, Grayson W. Recent advances in bioreactors for cell-based therapies. F1000Res. 2018;**7**:517. DOI: 10.12688/f1000research.12533.1. pii: F1000 Faculty Rev

[6] Nick C. The US Biosimilars Act: Challenges facing regulatory approval. Pharmaceutical Medicine. 2012;**26**(3):145-152. DOI: 10.1007/bf03262388

[7] Camacho LH, Frost CP, Abella E, Morrow PK, Whittaker S. Biosimilars 101: Considerations for U.S. oncologists in clinical practice. Cancer Medicine. 2014;**3**(4):889-899. DOI: 10.1002/cam4.258

[8] Lamanna WC, Holzmann J, Cohen HP, Guo X, Schweigler M, Stangler T, Seidl A, Schiestl M. Maintaining consistent quality and clinical performance of biopharmaceuticals. Expert Opinion on Biological Therapy. 2018;**18**(4):369-379. DOI: 10.1080/14712598.2018.1421169

[9] Strati P, Jain N, O'Brien S. Chronic lymphocytic leukemia: Diagnosis and treatment. Mayo Clinic Proceedings. 2018;**93**(5):651-664. DOI: 10.1016/j.mayocp.2018.03.002

[10] Marr KA, Datta K, Mehta S, Ostrander DB, Rock M, Francis J, Feldmesser M. Urine antigen detection as an aid to diagnose invasive aspergillosis. Clinical Infectious Diseases. 2018. DOI: 10.1093/cid/ciy326. [Epub ahead of print]

[11] Phuong NH, Kwak C, Heo CK, Cho EW, Yang J, Poo H. Development and characterization of monoclonal antibodies against nucleoprotein for diagnosis of influenza A virus. Journal of Microbiology and Biotechnology. 2018;**28**(5):809-815. DOI: 10.4014/jmb.1801.01002

[12] Chen YC, Cheng HF, Yang YC, Yeh MK. Nanotechnologies applied in biomedical vaccines. In: Stanciu SG, editor. Micro and Nanotechnologies for Biotechnology. Rijeka, Croatia: InTech; 2016. pp. 85-105. DOI: 10.5772/63453

[13] Chen YC, Cheng HF, Yang YC, Yeh MK. Biotechnologies applied in biomedical vaccines. In: Afrin F, Hemeg H, Ozbak H, editors. Vaccine. Rijeka, Croatia: InTech; 2017. pp. 97-110. DOI: 10.5772/intechopen.69547

[14] Das SK, Menezes ME, Bhatia S, Wang XY, Emdad L, Sarkar D, Fisher PB. Gene therapies for cancer: Strategies, challenges and successes. Journal of Cellular Physiology. 2015;**230**(2):259-271. DOI: 10.1002/jcp.24791

[15] Bai Y, Gong H, Li H, Vu GP, Lu S, Liu F. Oral delivery of RNase P ribozymes by *Salmonella* inhibits viral infections in mice. Proceedings of the National Academy of Sciences of the United States of America. 2011;**108**(8):3222-3227. DOI: 10.1073/pnas.1014975108

[16] Gan WB, Grutzendler J, Wong WT, Wong RO, Lichtman JW. Multicolor "DiOlistic" labeling of the nervous system using lipophilic dye combinations. Neuron. 2000;**27**(2):219-225. DOI: 10.1016/S0896-6273(00)00031-3

[17] Guo W, Guo Y, Tang S, Qu H, Zhao H. Dendritic cell-Ewing's sarcoma cell hybrids enhance antitumor immunity. Clinical Orthopaedics and Related Research. 2008;**466**(9):2176-2183. DOI: 10.1007/s11999-008-0348-7

[18] Stewart MP, Sharei A, Ding X, Sahay G, Langer R, Jensen KF. *In vitro* and strategies for intracellular delivery. Nature. 2016;**538**(7624):183-192. DOI: 10.1038/nature19764

[19] Oggu GS, Sasikumar S, Reddy N, Ella KKR, Rao CM, Bokara KK. Gene delivery approaches for mesenchymal stem cell therapy: Strategies to increase efficiency and specificity. Stem Cell Reviews. 2017;**13**(6):725-740. DOI: 10.1007/s12015-017-9760-2

[20] Xiao Q, Min T, Ma S, Hu L, Chen H, Lu D. Intracellular generation of single-strand template increases the knock-in efficiency by combining CRISPR/Cas9 with AAV. Molecular Genetics and Genomics. 2018;**293**(4):1051-1060. DOI: 10.1007/s00438-018-1437-2

[21] Finn JD, Smith AR, Patel MC, Shaw L, Youniss MR, van Heteren J, Dirstine T, Ciullo C, Lescarbeau R, Seitzer J, Shah RR, Shah A, Ling D, Growe J, Pink M, Rohde E, Wood KM, Salomon WE, Harrington WF, Dombrowski C, Strapps WR, Chang Y, Morrissey DV. A

single administration of CRISPR/Cas9 lipid nanoparticles achieves robust and persistent *in vivo* genome editing. Cell Reports. 2018;**22**(9):2227-2235. DOI: 10.1016/j.celrep.2018.02.014

[22] Lau CH, Suh Y. *In vivo* genome editing in animals using AAV-CRISPR system: Applications to translational research of human disease. F1000Res. 2017;**6**:2153. DOI: 10.12688/f1000research.11243.1

[23] Sipp D, Caulfield T, Kaye J, Barfoot J, Blackburn C, Chan S, De Luca M, Kent A, McCabe C, Munsie M, Sleeboom-Faulkner M, Sugarman J, van Zimmeren E, Zarzeczny A, Rasko JEJ. Marketing of unproven stem cell-based interventions: A call to action. Science Translational Medicine. 2017;**9**(397):pii: eaag0426. DOI: 10.1126/scitranslmed.aag0426

[24] Declerck P, Farouk-Rezk M, Rudd PM. Biosimilarity versus manufacturing change: Two distinct concepts. Pharmaceutical Research. 2016;**33**(2):261-268. DOI: 10.1007/s11095-015-1790-3

[25] Epstein MS, Ehrenpreis ED, Kulkarni PM. FDA-Related Matters Committee of the American College of Gastroenterology. Biosimilars: The need, the challenge, the future: The FDA perspective. The American Journal of Gastroenterology. 2014;**109**(12):1856-1859. DOI: 10.1038/ajg.2014.151

[26] Dougherty MK, Zineh I, Christl L. Perspectives on the current state of the biosimilar regulatory pathway in the United States. Clinical Pharmacology and Therapeutics. 2018;**103**(1):36-38. DOI: 10.1002/cpt.909

[27] Terson J, Budlong H, Affeldt T, Skiermont K, Kyllo G, Heaton A. Biosimilar products in the modern U.S. health care and regulatory landscape. Journal of Managed Care & Specialty Pharmacy. 2017;**23**(12):1255-1259. DOI: 10.18553/jmcp.2017.23.12.1255

Section 2

Characteristic

Chapter 2

Characterization of Biopharmaceuticals Focusing on Antibody Therapeutics

Woojeong Kim, Kui Hyun Kang and Jung-Keun Suh

Additional information is available at the end of the chapter

http://dx.doi.org/10.5772/intechopen.79107

Abstract

Biopharmaceuticals are highly complex molecules and also require high quality for safety and efficacy in human uses. For well-characterized products, the desired level of quality should be monitored and controlled during the manufacturing processes. A series of workflow for analytical characterization should be applied for product quality throughout those processes. In this chapter, several analytical techniques are introduced for assessing characteristics of biopharmaceuticals focusing on monoclonal antibodies (mAbs). Analytical characterization for primary structure was performed by mass spectrometry (MS), and assessment of post-translational modifications (PTMs) was done by conventional approaches. The analytical assessments were also done by multi-attribute method (MAM) approach using mass spectrometer (MS), and the performance of MAM was compared to conventional approaches.

Keywords: biopharmaceutical, analytical characterization, primary structure, mass spectrometry, post-translational modification (PTM), multi-attribute method (MAM)

1. Introduction

Biopharmaceuticals can be defined as protein drugs that are produced by recombinant DNA technology, such as hormones, enzymes, monoclonal antibodies, and fusion proteins used for therapeutic or diagnostic purposes [1]. The first biopharmaceutical, insulin, was introduced in 1982 [2], and since then, over 250 biopharmaceutical products are authorized for marketing in the two major regions, United States of America (USA) and Europe (EU). Those products can be classified into monoclonal antibodies (mAb), hormones, growth factors, vaccines, cytokines, blood factors, and others [3]. This trend with increasing number of biopharmaceuticals on the market results in gaining interest for drug development industry, and biopharmaceuticals are considered as fast growing and promising area for drug development [3–6].

The approval of mAb-related products is dramatically increased in the recent years [6, 7]. Over 90 mAb-related products are approved by European Medicines Agency (EMA) and US Food and Drug Administration (FDA). Those can be classified into mAb, Fc-fusion, Fab, antibody-drug conjugate (ADC), bispecific mAb (bsAb), and bispecific T cell engager (BiTE). Among them, mAbs are the major product, consisting of 77% of total. Others represent rest 23% of total, Fc-fusion (12%), ADC (5%), Fab (3%), bsAb (2%), and BiTE (1%), respectively. After the first approval of full-length mAb in 1998, mAbs are major product in the biopharmaceutical industry. This increasing number gives high revenue for pharmaceutical companies, and seven mAb-related products are positioned in top 10 drugs in the world, 2017, including Humira, Enbrel, Rituxan, Remicade, AVASTIN, Herceptin, and Lantus [8].

Mylotarg is the first approved ADC in 2000, which combined a mAb targeting leukemic blast cells with a bacterial toxin (calicheamicin) [7, 9]. ADC is a complex generated between a mAb and small molecule or a peptide, and mAb gives the selective delivery for targeting of cytotoxic drugs [1, 9–11]. Since the first approval, four additional ADC products are approved in Europe and USA. bsAb has two different antigen binding sites recognizing two different epitopes in a single mAb, and this dual specificity gives more specific targeting and higher efficacy [12–14]. Currently, three bsAbs are approved by EMA or US FDA. The first bsAb, Removab, was approved in 2009 but voluntarily withdrawn in 2013. Fc-fusion proteins are fusions of the IgG Fc domain with a desired linked protein, enhancing pharmacokinetic properties (serum half-life) and pharmacodynamics properties (ADCC and CDC) [6, 15]. Following the first approval of Fc-fusion protein, Enbrel in 1998, eight Fc-fusion proteins are authorized for the marketing in the region of Europe and USA.

Biosimilars, known as follow-on biologics, which follow termination of patent protection of original biopharmaceutical products, are developed and approved since 2006. Following the first approval from EMA, over 35 biosimilars are authorized for the European market and over 20 biosimilars are approved from FDA since 2015 [16–18]. A biosimilar is a biological product that is highly similar to and has no clinically meaningful differences from an existing FDA-approved reference product in terms of safety, purity, and potency (safety and effectiveness) [19]. Structural and clinical similarities are to be proven for the biosimilar authorization.

Biopharmaceuticals are highly complex molecules compared to small molecule drugs and should be monitored and controlled during the manufacturing processes for well-characterized products [20–22]. The characterization of biopharmaceuticals is challenging, which utilize the state-of-the-art technology to meet the international harmonized guidelines, Q5E and Q6B [23, 24]. For proper characterization, critical quality attributes (CQAs) have to be defined and evaluated that may impact on safety, purity, and potency. CQA is defined by ICHQ8(R2) as a physical, chemical, biological, or microbiological property of characteristic that should be within an appropriate limit, range, or distribution to ensure the desired product quality [25].

Within this chapter, methodologies for in-depth physicochemical characterization are introduced for recombinant biopharmaceuticals mainly focused on mAbs. Analytical characterization for primary structure was performed by mass spectrometry, and assessment of post-translational modifications (PTMs) was done with conventional and multi-attribute method (MAM) approaches. The performance of MAM was compared to conventional approach.

http://dx.doi.org/10.5772/intechopen.79107

2. Structural characterization for identity

2.1. Intact mass determination of mAb

The molecular weight of a protein is an important parameter in the physicochemical properties of the protein. MS with high resolution and accuracy, such as matrix-assisted laser desorption ionization time-of-flight (MALDI-TOF) or electrospray ionization quadrupole time-of-flight (ESI-QTOF), has become a reliable and sensitive technique for proteins and peptides to determine the molecular weight [26, 27]. Other high resolution mass spectrometers, Fourier transform ion cyclotron resonance (FTICR) and orbitrap MS, have been recently used for the intact mass analysis [28–30]. The workflow of ESI was further extended to native MS, having the capability to investigate intact mAb for structural analysis and heterogeneities from PTM [31, 32]. Applying intact mass analysis, it not only gives molecular mass of the intact protein for comparison with the theoretical mass but also provides quick information about primary structure of protein or sequence variants, such as isoforms, truncation, mutations, addition of signal sequences, or PTMs including glycosylations [31–33].

ESI-QTOF is widely used for measuring intact mass because of high resolution, mass accuracy, and easy connection to high performance liquid chromatography (HPLC) for online analysis [34]. ESI produces multiply charged ions, and those ions can be deconvoluted for molecular mass of proteins [34]. Typical results of mass determination for mAbs, bevacizumab, rituximab, and trastuzumab using ESI-QTOF are shown in **Figure 1**. MS spectra in inset of **Figure 1** show multiply charged ions characterized by ESI-spectrum, a number of peaks corresponding a statistical distribution of different charge states. The accuracy was less than 50 ppm, providing tools for the identification of PTMs, glycosylation, C-terminal Lysine deletion (ΔK), or Gln/Glu cyclization (pE) (**Figure 1**).

2.2. Subunit mass determination of mAb

Subunits or fragments of mAbs can be obtained by reduction of disulfide bonds or proteolysis to reduce complexities for large size mAbs [36, 37]. Chemical reduction of mAb's disulfide bond generates free heavy chains and light chains, having ~50 kDa and ~25 kDa molecular mass, respectively. Recently, a new protease IdeS (Immunoglobulin G-degrading enzyme of *Streptococcus pyogenes*), specifically cleaving between the two consecutive glycine residues of the hinge region, has been described for mAb fragmentations [29, 37–39]. IdeS treatment of

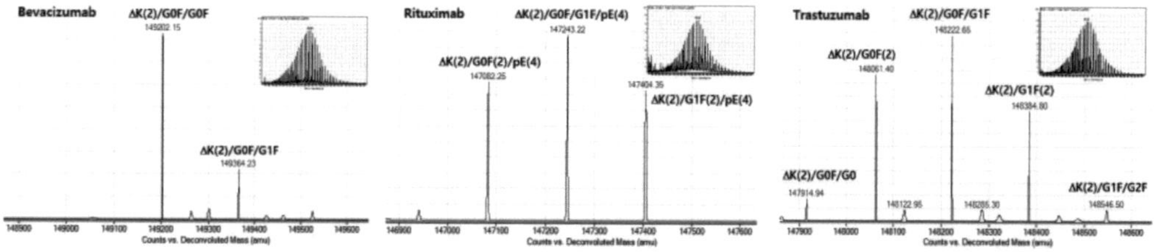

Figure 1. Intact mass of mAbs determined by deconvolution using ESI-QTOF. Inserts show charge envelope having multiply charged ions. Glycan structures (G0F, G1F, and G2F) were adapted from [35]. ΔK: C-terminal Lys deletion and pE: pyro-glutamate.

mAbs with subsequent chemical reduction generates three subunits, Fd, LC, and Fc/2, having ~25 kDa molecular mass. Those subunits can be separated by reverse phase (RP)-HPLC analysis and be analyzed using online MS analysis. A typical example of IdeS treatment of mAb is shown in **Figure 2**. The subunits of rituximab were generated by IdeS digestion with subsequent chemical reduction and separated by RP-HPLC. The molecular masses of the subunits were measured by online ESI-QTOF. Three subunits from IdeS-digested rituximab, Fc/2, LC, and Fd, were clearly separated on the chromatogram of RP-HPLC (**Figure 2**). The deconvolution of ESI-QTOF spectra for subunits gives molecular mass information (**Figure 3**, inset). The molecular masses for Fc/2, LC, or Fd subunits were 25.4, 23.0, or 25.3 kDa, respectively. This not only provides tools for N-glycan profiling but also allows identification of PTMs such as C-terminal Lys deletion and cyclization of N-terminal glutamine (**Figure 2**).

2.3. Peptide mapping of mAb

The peptide mapping is a gold standard for biopharmaceutical characterization not only as an identity test but also to demonstrate the integrity of disulfide bonds [40–43]. This analytical method provides detailed information of primary structure for a given protein and enables the control of the protein sequence down to the level of single amino acids by coupling with mass spectrometry [44–46]. Based on the analysis of peptide mapping, it is possible to confirm genetic stability (correct translation), identify post-translation modification, and demonstrate the integrity of disulfide bonds [47–50].

Peptide mapping was carried out by digesting protein samples with endoprotease, such as trypsin, and subsequent separation of peptide fragments by RP-HPLC. The peptide fragments are then monitored by UV absorption and identified by MS. Prior to protease digestion, denaturation of the test protein with known concentration is needed to ensure complete digestion. The measured absorbance of a protein sample solution is used to calculate the concentration from its absorptivity at 280 nm (A280) either experimentally determined or empirically calculated [22, 51]. Denaturation can be done using chaotropic reagent, urea, SDS, guanidine, or

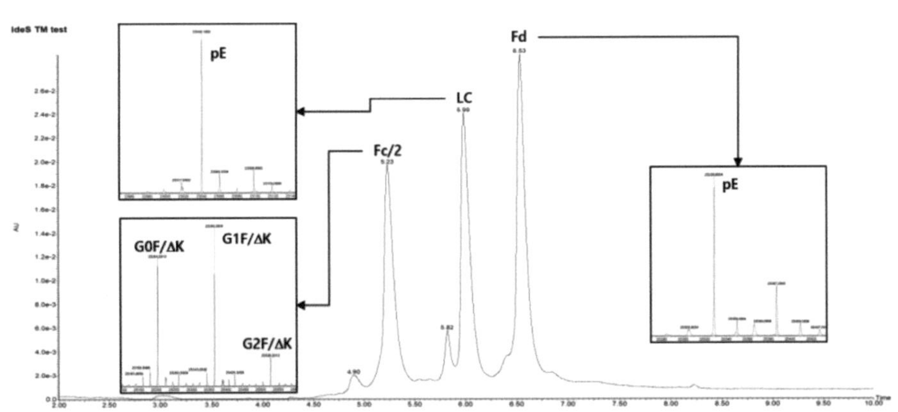

Figure 2. UV chromatogram of RP-HPLC for IdeS-digested Rituximab. Three subunits (Fc/2, LC, and Fd) are resolved on the chromatogram, and deconvoluted monoisotopic masses for each subunit are shown in insets. Glycan structures (G0F, G1F, and G2F) were adapted from [35]. ΔK: C-terminal Lys deletion and pE: pyro-glutamate.

http://dx.doi.org/10.5772/intechopen.79107

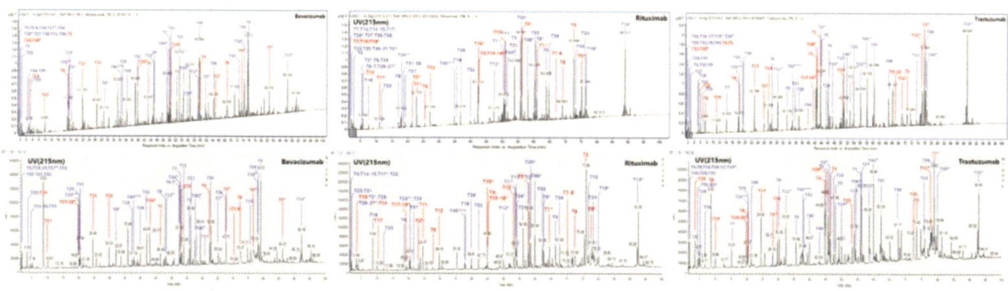

Figure 3. Identified peptides of three mAbs, bevacizumab, rituximab, and trastuzumab, by peptide mapping analysis using QTOF (Top) or Orbitrap (Bottom). Blue: peptides from heavy chain, Red: peptides from light chain. *Alkylated peptides, **N-glycopeptide, ***C-terminal Lys deleted peptide, and ^pyroglutamic acid Q N-term.

acid-labile surfactant, RapiGest [50, 51]. Denatured proteins are further reduced and alkylated. Reduction of disulfide bonds can be done with dithiothreitol (DTT), 2-Mercapto-ethanol, or tris(2-carboxyethyl)phosphine (TCEP) and alkylation with iodoacetamide or iodoacetic acid to prevent free cysteine groups after reduction [52, 53].

Many proteases are available for protein digestion, each having their own characteristics in terms of specificity, efficiency, and optimum digestion conditions [54, 55]. Trypsin is the most commonly used protease for peptide mapping analysis because it has a well-defined specificity. It hydrolyzes only the peptide bonds in which the carbonyl group is followed either by an arginine (Arg) or lysine (Lys) residue and the cleavage will not occur if proline is positioned on the carboxyl side of Lys or Arg [56, 57].

After digestion, resulting peptides are separated by RP-HPLC, detected by UV-absorption, and identified by mass spectrometry. The identity of the samples was confirmed by comparing the peak profile taking into account the number of detected peaks, retention times, and peak areas of the individual peaks. Furthermore, the measured masses of the found tryptic peptides were compared to the theoretical masses calculated from the amino acid sequence to verify the correct identification of the single peptides. Recently, the development of ultra-high performance chromatography (UHPLC) and sub-2 μm solid core particle columns leads to improve peak resolution and width, resulting in enhancing efficiency, sensitivity, and reproducibility for peptide identification [58–63]. To identify peptides with MS, peptides need to be transferred into gas phase by ionization such as ESI or MALDI [64, 65]. ESI is commonly used for peptide mapping in combination with HPLC separations. The hybrid mass instruments, Q-Orbitrap and QTOF with ESI ionization, are routinely used for peptide mapping of mAbs [66, 67].

Typical results of peptide mapping of bevacizumab, rituximab, and trastuzumab are shown in **Figure 3**. For the peptide mapping analysis, protein samples were digested with trypsin, and the resulting peptides were separated using RP-UHPLC, detected by UV-absorption, and identified by online ESI-QTOF or Orbitrap (Fusion). Peptide map analysis covers the full sequence of mAbs, with the exception of the small polar peptides, giving over 98% coverage for overall sequences. Along with the intact peptides, modified peptides were also identified, such as glycopeptides, C-terminal Lys deleted peptides, and peptides with Gln cyclization.

2.4. Disulfide bond identification for mAb

Protein disulfide bonds are produced by the covalent bonding of two thiol groups between cysteine amino acids. They are essential for structural and functional roles of proteins and give stability of proteins [68, 69]. The number of disulfide bonds and their positions are a critical attribute for biopharmaceuticals to ensure safety and efficacy [70, 71]. Peptide mapping coupled with LC-MS offers fast and accurate workflow for characterizing disulfide bonds of proteins. The typical workflow for identifying disulfide bonds in proteins is done by peptide mapping with the conditions of reduced and non-reduced digestion, and these two conditions are compared using LC-MS and LC-MS/MS [72, 73].

The typical result of disulfide bond identification for trastuzumab is shown in **Figure 4**. It is known that trastuzumab (IgG1) has 32 cysteine residues, which are cross-linked by four interchain disulfide bonds (two set of a disulfide bond between heavy and light chains, two between heavy chains) and two set of six intrachain disulfide bonds [74]. When trastuzumab is compared for tryptic map between reduced and non-reduced condition, 16 tryptic peptides (T) having cysteine residues (for heavy chain (H)— H:T2 (Cys22), H:T11 (Cys96), H:T14 (Cys147), H:T15 (Cys203), H:T19 (Cys223), H:T20 (Cys229, Cys232), H:C27(Cys229, Cys232), H:T22 (Cys264), H:T28 (Cys324), H:T36 (Cys370), and H:T41 (Cys428); for light chain (L)—L:T2 (Cys23), L:T7 (Cys88), L:T11 (Cys134), L:T18 (Cys194), and L:T20 (Cys214)) are expected under reduced condition as shown in **Figure 4**. Under non-reduced condition, six peptides linked by an intra-chain disulfide bond (H:T2 = H:T11, H:T14 = H:T15, H:T22 = H:T28, H:T36 = H:T41, L:T2 = L:T7, and L:T11 = L:T18), a peptide linked by a disulfide bond between heavy and light chains (L:T19-20 = H:T19), and a peptide linked by two disulfide bonds between heavy chains (H:T20 = H:T20) are generated as shown in **Figure 4**.

Collision-induced dissociation (CID) for disulfide-bonded peptide usually generates b and y ions from two individual peptides as shown in **Figure 5**, requiring side-by-side comparison between reduced and non-reduced peptide map [75]. Electron-transfer dissociation (ETD) usually generates disulfide-bonded fragment ions from both peptides, simultaneously detecting disulfide-bonded fragments and disulfide-bonded precursor peptide and simplifying the workflow for CID fragmentation without parallel side-by-side comparison [76]. The data-independent MSE approach collects mass data of precursors and fragments of eluting peptide from protein digests in an unbiased manner for peptide mapping and disulfide bond analyses [77, 78]. An example of disulfide bond analysis using MSE is shown in **Figure 5**. The MSE spectrum not only contains b and y ions from the two individual peptides (H:T2 and H:T11)

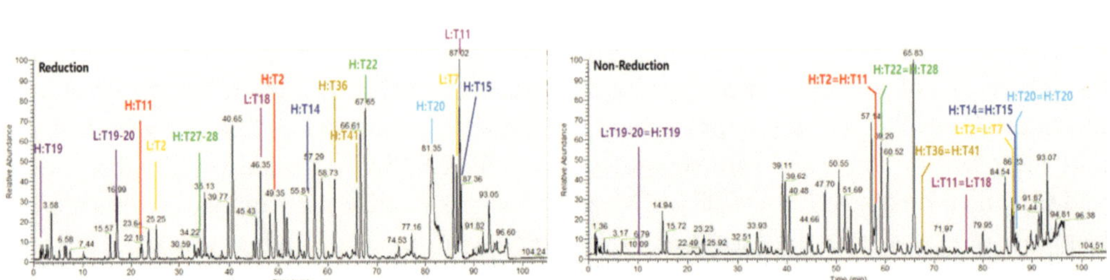

Figure 4. Identification of disulfide bonds for trastuzumab by peptide mapping under reduced (left) and non-reduced (right) tryptic digestions.

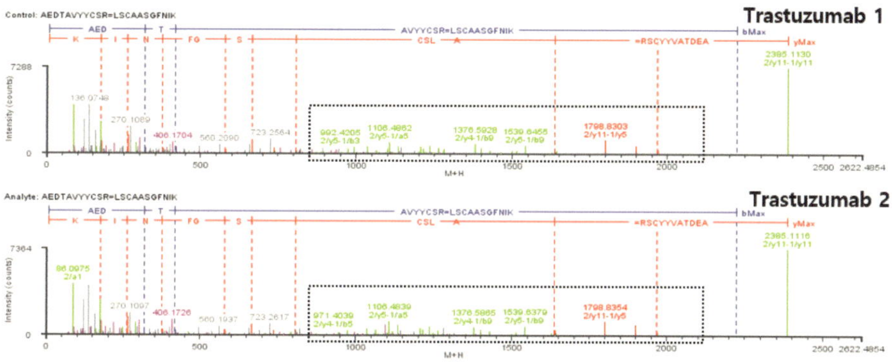

Figure 5. Fragmentation of disulfide-bonded peptide (H:T2 = H:T11) from trastuzumab by MSE approach using CID.

but also has ions corresponding to disulfide-bonded fragments from both peptides shown (H:T2 = H:T11) in dotted box in **Figure 5**.

3. Post-translational modification (PTM)

PTMs can be classified into two major classes, enzymatic and chemical modifications. Enzymatic modifications are defined as enzyme-catalyzed processing of proteins after translation by kinases, phosphatases, proteases, transferases, ligases, etc. [79]. Most common PTMs in this class are glycosylation, disulfide bond formation, and proteolytic cleavage of the protein. Chemical modifications are generated during upstream and downstream processing, formulation, and storage, including oxidation, deamidation, isomerization, glycation, and Gln/Glu cyclization [80]. Those PTMs can affect activity, stability, and immunogenicity and thus must be well-characterized, controlled, and monitored during development processes [20, 21, 81]. Physicochemical and biological analyses are required for monitoring those PTMs [82–86]. Peptide mapping approach is one of those method capable for the site-specific identification and quantitation of various PTMs. Recently multi-attribute method (MAM) has been developed as MS-based method that is able to identify and quantify several attribute at once [48, 87, 88]. The conventional methods such as hydrophilic interaction chromatography (HILIC) for oligosaccharide analysis, cation-exchange (CEX) chromatography, and capillary electrophoresis sodium dodecyl sulfate (CE-SDS) can be replaced by MAM approach (**Table 1**).

3.1. Glycosylation of mAb

Glycosylation is a major PTM, influencing protein folding and conformation. Thus, heterogeneity due to glycosylation may affect the bioactivity [89, 90]. Most mAbs have a single N-glycosylation site in Fc subunit (e.g., heavy chain N300), although some mAbs may have an additional glycosylation site in Fab subunit. Glycosylation on mAbs is known to affect their effector functions such as complement activation, antibody-dependent cell cytotoxicity (ADCC), cytotoxic endocytosis of immune complexes leading to antigen presentation, and inhibition of B lymphocytes, monocytes, and basophils [90–93].

Attribute	Description	Current workflow	Future development
N-term sequences	Identity	Edman Degradation	Multi-attribute method (MAM)
N-term variants	Gln/Glu cyclization	CEX-HPLC	
C-term variants	C-term Lys deletion	CEX-HPLC	
Charge variants	Deamidation/Isomerization	CEX-HPLC	
Clips	Fragment	CE-SDS	
Glycans	Glycosylation	HILIC	

HILIC: hydrophilic interaction chromatography, CEX-HPLC: cation-exchange high performance liquid chromatography, and CE-SDS: capillary electrophoresis-sodium dodecyl sulfate.

Table 1. MS-based MAM for attribute control compared to current workflow.

Glycan profiling can be done by releasing glycan moieties from mAbs using PNGase F and cleaving the linkage between GlcNAc and Asn. The released N-glycans are done by fluorescent labeling and subsequently analyzed using HPLC with fluorescence detector (FLD) coupled to MS instrument [94]. The recent development of HILIC and ultra-high pressure liquid chromatography with sub-2 μm amide-bonded stationary phases enables to separate labeled N-glycans with high resolution [95–97]. The typical result of N-glycan profiling is shown in **Figure 6**. Based on the detected mass by MS analysis, potential structures are all assigned for each peak, and the relative contents are calculated for the assigned structures from FLD detection (**Table 2**). G0F and G1F are major glycans on trastuzumab. The contents of afucosylated N-glycans are around 9.9% and that of high mannose type N-glycan around 1.7% of total. Sialylated N-glycans are not detected on this analysis.

For MAM approach for glycan profile, glycopeptides were identified by peptide mapping of mAb, trastuzumab. Different N-glycans were identified on the N300 of the H:T25 peptide (EEQYNSTYR), such as G0F-GlcNac, G0, G0F, Man5, G1, G1F, G2F, and G2F + 1SA. Intact peptide without N-glycan was also detected. **Figure 7** shows the identified glycopeptide from peptide mapping analysis.

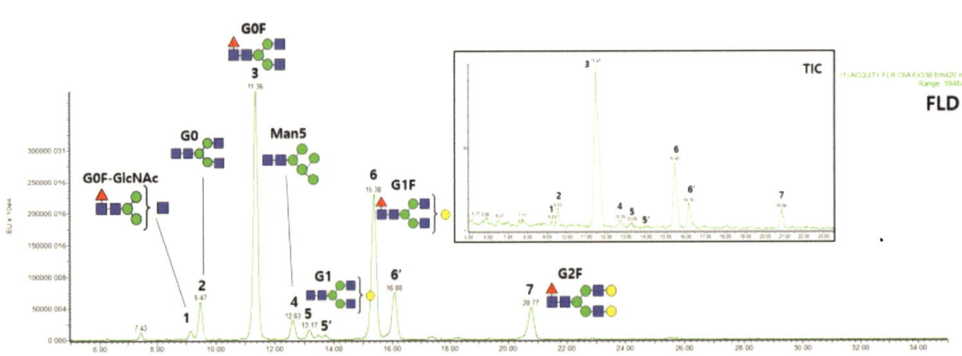

Figure 6. N-glycan profiling of mAb, trastuzumab, using HILIC-FLD-MS. Total ion chromatogram (TIC) and FLD chromatogram of N-glycans are shown. Inset represents TIC. Glycan structures (G0F, G1F, G2F, or etc.) were adapted from [35].

Peak	1	2	3	4	5 and 5′	6 and 6′	7
Glycan	G0F-GlcNAc	G0	G0F	Man5	G1	G1F	G2F
Relative content (%)	0.48 ± 0.09	6.48 ± 0.96	43.58 ± 1.81	1.66 ± 0.22	1.71 ± 0.11	39.10 ± 1.73	6.98 ± 0.49

Glycan structures (G0F, G1F, G2F, or etc.) were adapted from [35].

Table 2. N-glycan profiling of mAb, trastuzumab, determined by HILIC-FLD-MS.

Based on MS/MS analysis, potential structures are assigned for glycopeptide peak. The relative contents are calculated from XIC for the assigned structures (**Table 3**). The mass accuracy was determined by Eq. (1) and less than ±5 ppm. G0F and G1F are major glycans on trastuzumab. The contents of afucosylated N-glycans are around 12.2% and that of high mannose type N-glycan around 6.42% of total. A sialylated N-glycan was detected less than 1%.

Calculation of error for determined peptide by MS is shown in Eq. (1)

$$\text{Error (ppm)} = [(\text{Determined Mass-Calculated Mass})/\text{Determined Mass}] \times 10^6 \quad (1)$$

To compare N-glycan profiling results between HILIC and MAM approaches, the relative contents for each N-glycan between two approaches are visualized and a linear regression analysis was performed. The results are shown in **Figure 8**. The relative amounts of G0, G0F, and G1F are slightly higher in HILIC than MAM but those of Man5 and G2F are higher in MAM than HILIC (**Figure 9**). From the regression analysis, the slope was 0.816, intercept was 2.307, and correlation coefficient was 0.958, which indicates a correlation between HILIC and MAM approaches.

3.2. Deamidation and isomerization of mAb

The major cause of charge variants in mAbs is deamidation and isomerization [98–100]. Asparagine (Asn) and glutamine (Gln) are susceptible to deamidation, but glutamine is deamidated at a much lower rate than that of asparagine [101–103]. Deamidation of Asn is

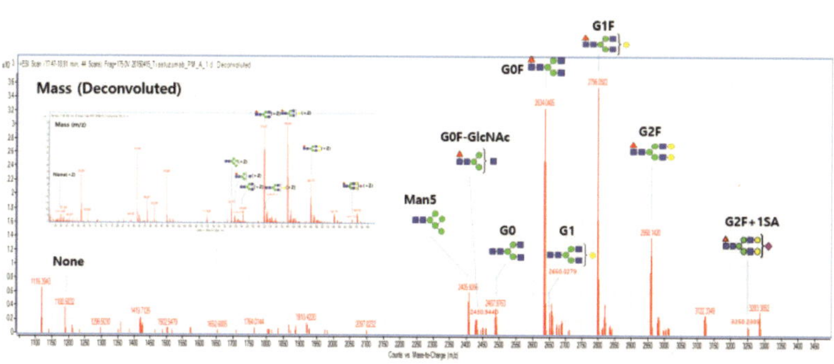

Figure 7. Glycopeptide having different N-glycans identified by peptide mapping analysis of trastuzumab. Inset represents MS1 spectrum before deconvolution. Glycan structures (G0F, G1F, G2F, or etc.) were adapted from [35].

Peptide	Number	Glycan attached	Calculated mass (Da)	Determined mass (Da)	Error (ppm)	Relative content (%)
EEQYNSTYR	H:T25		1188.5047	1188.502	−2.27	2.18 ± 0.06
EEQYNSTYR	H:T25**	Man5	2404.9276	2404.9249	−1.12	6.42 ± 0.27
EEQYNSTYR	H:T25**	G0F-GlcNAc	2429.9592	2429.9531	−2.51	1.23 ± 0.04
EEQYNSTYR	H:T25**	G0	2486.9807	2486.9744	−2.53	3.21 ± 0.19
EEQYNSTYR	H:T25**	G0F	2633.0386	2633.0395	0.34	36.25 ± 0.68
EEQYNSTYR	H:T25**	G1	2649.0335	2649.031	−0.94	2.56 ± 0.18
EEQYNSTYR	H:T25**	G1F	2795.0914	2795.093	0.57	34.05 ± 0.80
EEQYNSTYR	H:T25**	G2F	2957.1443	2957.1398	−1.52	13.25 ± 0.85
EEQYNSTYR	H:T25**	G2F + 1SA	3248.2397	3248.2295	−3.14	0.86 ± 0.00

Glycan structures (G0F, G1F, G2F, or etc.) were adapted from Ref. [35]. **: N-glycosylated Peptide.

Table 3. N-glycan profiling of mAb, trastuzumab, determined by MAM approach.

a non-enzymatic process, converting Asn to a 5-ringed cyclic succinimide intermediate that is hydrolyzed to form a mixture of isoaspartic acid (isoAsp or isoD) and aspartic acid (Asp) [104]. Isomerization follows the same mechanism of deamidation but occurs at aspartic acid (Asp) residues to form iso-Asp through the succinimide intermediate [105, 106]. This results in product heterogeneity and complicates manufacturing consistency [107]. Deamidation and isomerization are also known to have significant impact on in vitro potency, product heterogeneity, shelf-life stability, manufacturing consistency, and yield [108–110].

CEX-HPLC and isoelectric focusing (IEF) have been successfully developed to investigate the charge variants due to deamidation and isomerization [111, 112]. Peptide mapping analysis

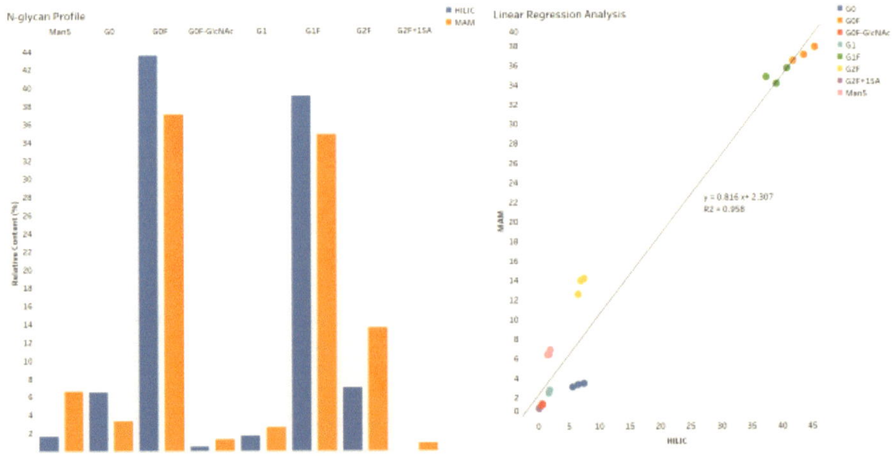

Figure 8. Glycan profiles determined by HILIC and MAM approaches.

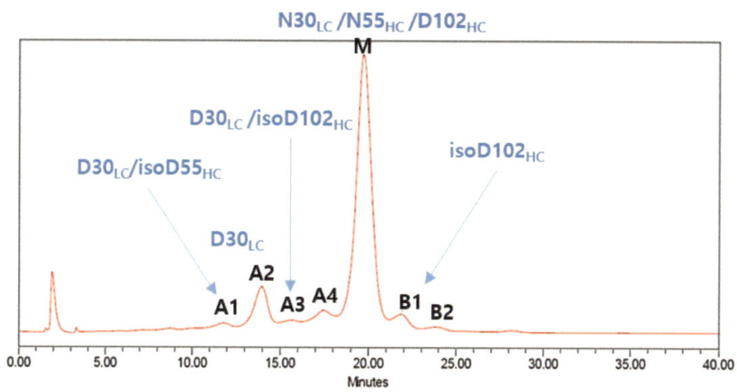

Figure 9. Profiling of charge variants from mAb, trastuzumab, by CEX-HPLC analysis. N: asparagine, D: aspartate, isoD: iso-aspartate, HC: heavy chain, and LC: light chain.

based on LC-MS/MS is commonly applied for identification of site and quantification of deamidation and isomerization, including the succinimide intermediated [113, 114].

CEX-HPLC can detect the occurrence of deamidation or C-terminal Lys deletion as well as glycosylation variants. The result of charge variant profiling for mAb, trastuzumab, is shown in **Figure 9**. Four acidic variants and two basic variants were detected on the CEX chromatogram. Each fraction for charge variants was collected, and the pooled fractions were further analyzed to characterize modification site by peptide mapping analysis. This analysis gives the structural information for each variant, and most of the charge variants are produced by deamidation and isomerization, localized on the CDR regions of mAb, trastuzumab (**Figure 9**).

UV detection of CEX chromatography allows to quantify charge variant peaks and the relative contents are calculated (**Table 4**). The content of major form without deamidation or isomerization on CDR regions is around 71.2%, that of acidic charge variants (A1-A4) are around 22.4%, and that of basic variants (B1-B2) is around 6.4% of total (**Table 4**).

Peak	N30(LC)	N55(HC)	D102(HC)	Relative content (%)
A1	D/N	isoD/N	D/D	0.24 ± 0.05
A2	D/N	N/N	D/D	10.60 ± 0.30
A3	D/N	N/N	isoD/D	3.89 ± 0.18
A4	N/N	N/N	D/D	7.68 ± 0.10
M	N/N	N/N	D/D	71.14 ± 0.58
B1	N/N	N/N	isoD/D	5.06 ± 0.26
B2	N/N	N/N	isoD/D	1.38 ± 0.05

N: asparagine, D: glutamate, isoD: iso-glutamate.

Table 4. The relative contents of charge variants identified by CEX analysis.

For MAM approach for charge variant profile including deamidation and isomerization, modified peptides were identified from peptide mapping analysis of mAb, trastuzumab. Deamidation on Asn30 of light chain was detected and isomerization on Asp102 of heavy chain was also detected by peptide mapping analysis using LC-MS/MS. However, deamination and isomerization on N55 of heavy chain were not detected. **Figure 10** shows the results of deamidation and isomerization on Asn30 of light chain and Asp102 of heavy chain, respectively.

Based on MS/MS analysis, peptide sequences are confirmed for intact and modified peptides. The relative contents are calculated from XIC for the intact and modified peptides (**Table 5**). The mass accuracy was determined by Eq. (1) and less than ±5 ppm. Isomerization on Asp102 of heavy chain was detected and its relative content was around 4.6% of total (**Table 5**). Intact and isomerized peptide has same molecular mass, and thus, it is not possible to distinguish from each other only by mass, but those peptides have different retention time on the chromatogram (**Figure 10**). Deamidation on Asn30 of light chain was detected and its relative content was around 7.7% of total (**Table 5**). Deamination and isomerization on N55 of heavy chain were not detected.

To compare profiling results of deamidation and isomerization between CEX and MAM approaches, the relative contents for each modified peptide between two approaches are visualized and a linear regression analysis was performed. The result from CEX contains information not from peptide levels but from full mAb, and thus CEX data were recalculated for the level of each amino acid comparable for MAM data. The results are shown in **Figure 11**. The relative amounts of deamidation and isomerization are very similar between CEX and MAM approaches (**Figure 11**). From the regression analysis, the slope was 1.038, intercept was 0.267, and correlation coefficient was 0.988, which indicates a very good correlation between HILIC and MAM approaches.

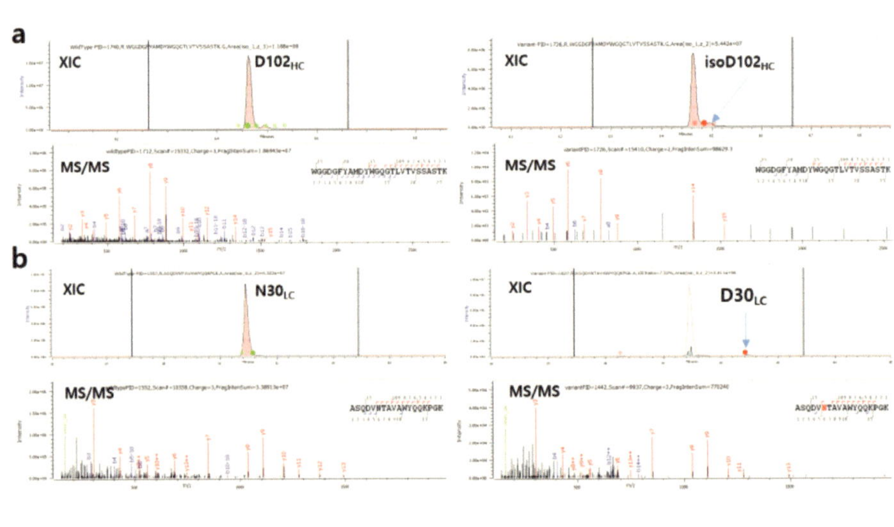

Figure 10. Isomerization on Asp102 of heavy chain (a) and deamidation on Asn30 of heavy chain (b). N: asparagine, D: aspartate, isoD: iso-aspartate, HC: heavy chain, LC: light chain.

http://dx.doi.org/10.5772/intechopen.79107

Peptide	Number	Change	Calculated mass (Da)	Mass (Da)	Error (ppm)	Relative content (%)
WGGDGFYAM DYWGQGTLV TVSSASTK	H:T12	D102	2783.2537	2783.2551	0.50	95.36 ± 0.28
WGG$_{iso}$DGFYAM DYWGQGTLV TVSSASTK	H:T12*	D102 to $_{iso}$D102	2783.2537	2783.2595	2.08	4.63 ± 0.28
IYPTNGYTR	H:T6	N55	1083.5349	1083.5345	−0.37	100
IYPT$_{iso}$DGYTR	H:T6*	N55 to $_{iso}$D55	1083.5349	—	—	0
ASQDVNTAV AWYQQKPGK	L:T3	N30	1989.9908	1989.9938	1.51	92.35 ± 0.24
ASQDVDTAV AWYQQKPGK	L:T3*	N30 to D30	1990.9749	1990.9774	1.26	7.70 ± 0.24

N: asparagine, D: aspartate, isoD: iso-aspartate, H: heavy chain, L: light chain, and T: tryptic peptide.
*: Deamidated or isomerized peptide.

Table 5. The relative contents of deamidation and isomerization identified by MAM analysis.

3.3. C-terminal Lys deletion of mAb

C-terminal Lys variants are clipped modification found at heavy chain C-terminus of mAbs produced in mammalian cell cultures, usually produced by proteolysis of endogenous carboxypeptidases during the manufacturing process [115, 116]. C-terminal Lys deletion has been known for no impact on antibody function, such as biologic activity, structural stability, pharmacokinetics, or bioavailability in rats [117]. However, there have been debates about impacts of C-terminal Lys deletion on Fc effector functions [117, 118].

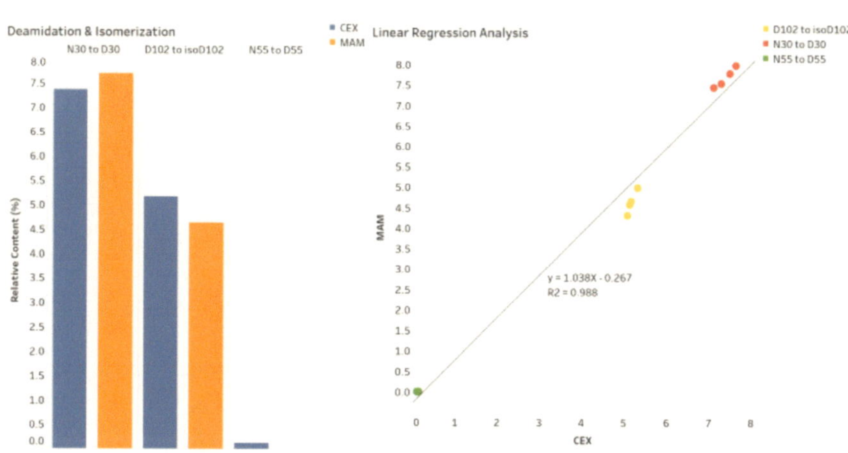

Figure 11. Profiles of deamidation and isomerization determined by CEX and MAM approaches. N: asparagine, D: aspartate, isoD: iso-aspartate, HC: heavy chain, and LC: light chain.

Because Lys residue is positively charged, leading to charge heterogeneity of mAb products. Thus, it is still a quality parameter for characterization. Due to charge variation, the modified and unmodified structures can be separated by CEX, IEF, and cIEF [117, 119]. Loss of the terminal Lys residue gives mass shift, which can be also detected and quantified by mass spectrometry [115, 118]. The modified structures can be separated and also identified from the unmodified structures by comparing the results from carboxypeptidase treatment [115, 120]. Carboxypeptidase treatment removes C-terminal Lys of mAbs and the disappeared peaks on the chromatogram can be identified as the unmodified variants [115, 120–122].

The typical results of CEX analysis are shown in **Figure 12**, which identify and quantify C-terminal Lys variants of mAb, adalimumab. Five acidic variants and three basic variants are detected (**Figure 12**). With the treatment of carboxypeptidase, all of the basic peaks were disappeared on the chromatogram (**Figure 12**, inset). Thus, those peaks are the unmodified peaks having C-terminal Lys.

UV detection of CEX chromatography allows to quantify C-terminal Lys variant peaks and the relative contents are calculated (**Table 6**). The content of major form is around 64.7%, that of C-terminal Lys variants on both heavy chains (A1-A4 and M) are around 77.5%, that of C-terminal Lys variants on one heavy chain (B1 and B2) are around 18.3%, and that of intact C-terminal Lys (B3) is around 4.1% of total (**Table 6**).

For MAM approach for C-terminal Lys variant profile, modified peptides were identified from peptide mapping analysis of mAb, adalimumab. **Figure 13** shows the results of C-terminal Lys variant of adalimumab. Based on MS/MS analysis, peptide sequences are confirmed for intact and modified peptides. XICs of confirmed peptides were determined and quantified. The mass accuracy was determined by Eq. (1) and less than ±5 ppm. C-terminal Lys variant was detected and its relative content was around 13% of total (**Table 7**).

To compare profiling results of C-terminal Lys variants between CEX and MAM approaches, the relative contents for each modified peptide between two approaches are visualized and a linear regression analysis was performed. The result from IEX contains information not from peptide levels but from full mAb, and thus, CEX data were recalculated for the level of each

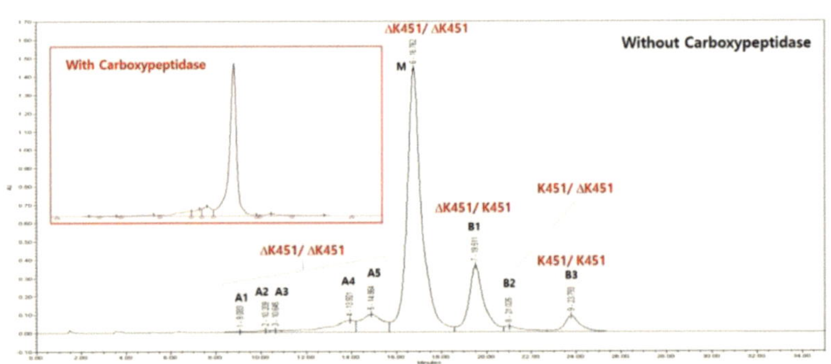

Figure 12. Profiling of C-terminal Lys variants from mAb, adalimumab, by CEX analysis. Inset represents the CEX chromatogram after carboxypeptidase treatment. K: Lys and ΔK: Lys deletion.

Peak	C-terminal structure of heavy chains	Relative content (%)
A1	Lys Deleted/Lys Deleted	0.10 ± 0.05
A2	Lys Deleted/Lys Deleted	0.54 ± 0.14
A3	Lys Deleted/Lys Deleted	0.29 ± 0.04
A4	Lys Deleted/Lys Deleted	5.52 ± 0.20
A5	Lys Deleted/Lys Deleted	6.422 ± 0.21
M	Lys Deleted/Lys Deleted	64.65 ± 0.34
B1	Lys Deleted/Intact Lys	16.55 ± 0.21
B2	Intact Lys/Lys Deleted	1.78 ± 0.12
B3	Intact Lys/Intact Lys	4.15 ± 0.09

A: acidic, M: major, B: basic.

Table 6. The relative contents of C-terminal Lys variants from adalimumab identified by IEX analysis.

amino acid comparable for MAM data. Along with adalimumab results, those of trastuzumab were also visualized. The results are shown in **Figure 14**. The relative amounts of C-terminal Lys variants from adalimumab and trastuzumab are very similar between CEX and MAM approaches (**Figure 14**). From the regression analysis for adalimumab and trastuzumab, the slope was 0.970, intercept was 2.935, and correlation coefficient was 0.998, which indicates a very good correlation between CEX and MAM approaches.

3.4. N-terminal cyclization of mAb

N-terminal cyclization (pyroGlu or pE) variants are generated by the rearrangement of Gln or Glu at the N-terminus of mAbs, which can be done by spontaneous or enzymatic reactions [123, 124]. The conversion rate from Gln to pyroGlus is much faster than that from Glu and nearly completed over 95% in mAbs having N-terminal Gln, which is known that this conversion occurs primarily in bioreactors [123]. The N-terminal cyclizations of mAbs converting Gln/Glu to pyroGlu do not impact on their structure, activity, in vivo clearance, and other pharmacokinetic properties [124].

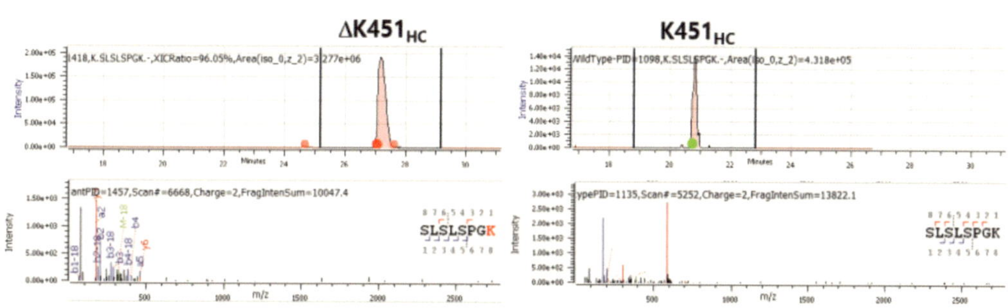

Figure 13. Identification of C-terminal Lys variant from adalimumab by peptide mapping analysis. K: Lys, ΔK: Lys deletion, and HC: heavy chain.

Peptide	Number	Modification	Calculated mass (Da)	Mass (Da)	Error (ppm)	Relative content (%)
SLSLSPGK	H:T40		787.4440	787.4434	−0.76	13.01 ± 0.38
SLSLSPG	H:T40*	K → ΔK	659.3489	659.3489	0.00	86.99 ± 0.38

K: Lys and Δ K: C-terminal Lys deletion. *: Deamidated or isomerized peptide.

Table 7. The relative contents of C-terminal Lys variants from adalimumab identified by MAM analysis.

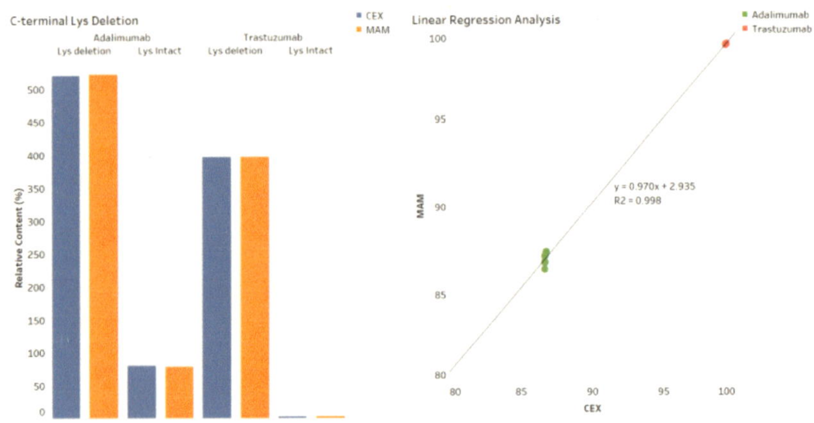

Figure 14. Profiles of C-terminal Lys variants for adalimumab and trastuzumab determined by CEX and MAM approaches.

The conversion from Gln to pyroGlu renders mAbs more acidic and the conversion from Glu to pyroGlu gives a basic shift. Thus, the N-terminal cyclization increases charge heterogeneity of mAb products, which can be detected by charge-based methods such as CEX, IEF, and cIEF. The conversion of Gln or Glu to pyroGlu gives a mass shift −17 or − 18 Da, respectively, compared to the unmodified peptide, and this can be assessed using peptide mapping and intact mass analysis by MS.

The typical results of CEX analysis are shown in **Figure 15**, which identify and quantify N-terminal cyclization variants of mAb, rituximab. On the chromatogram of rituximab, several acidic variants and two major basic variants are detected (**Figure 15**). Each fraction for basic charge variants was collected and the pooled fractions were further analyzed to characterize modification site by peptide mapping analysis. This analysis gives the structural information for each variant, and the basic variant (B2) are produced by N-terminal cyclization of light chain, rituximab (**Figure 16**).

UV detection of IEX chromatography allows to quantify this N-terminal cyclization variant and the relative content of it is calculated (**Table 8**). The content of major form is around 89.4% and that of N-terminal cyclization variant on a light chain is around 1.9% (**Table 8**).

For MAM approach for detecting and quantifying N-terminal cyclization of mAb, rituximab, the conversion from N-terminal Gln to pyroGlu was identified by peptide mapping analysis.

http://dx.doi.org/10.5772/intechopen.79107

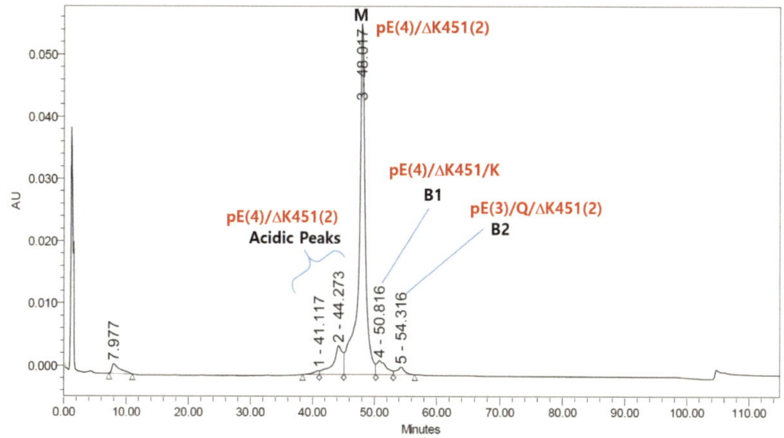

Figure 15. Profiling of N-terminal cyclization variant from mAb, rituximab, by IEX analysis. K: Lys, ΔK: Lys deletion, and pE: pyro-glutamate.

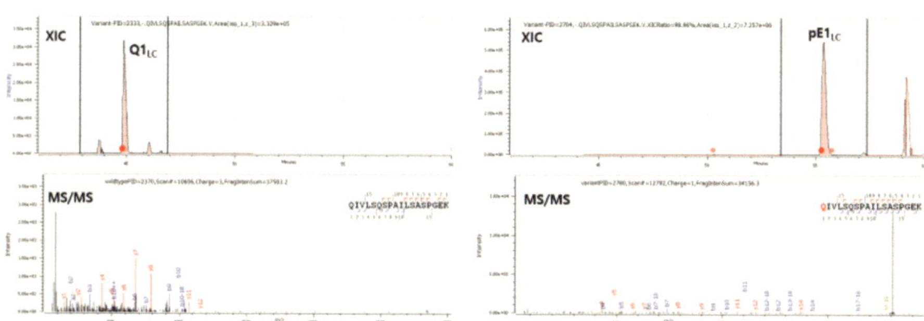

Figure 16. Identification of N-terminal cyclization variant from rituximab by peptide mapping analysis. Q: glutamine, pE: pyro-glutamate, and LC: light chain.

N-terminal cyclization on Gln1 of light chain was detected but N-terminal cyclization on Gln1 of heavy chain was not detected by peptide mapping analysis. **Figure 16** shows the results of N-terminal cyclization on Gln1 of light chain of mAb, rituximab.

Based on MS/MS analysis, peptide sequences are confirmed for intact and modified peptides. The relative contents are calculated from XIC for the intact and modified peptides. The mass accuracy was determined by Eq. (1) and less than ±5 ppm. N-terminal cyclization variant of light chain was detected and its relative content was around 99% of total (**Table 9**).

To compare profiling results of N-terminal cyclization variant between CEX and MAM approaches, the relative contents for each modified peptide between two approaches are compared and visualized. The relative amounts of N-terminal cyclization variant from rituximab are very similar between CEX and MAM approaches (**Figure 17**).

3.5. Other PTMs of mAb

Many other PTMs can be identified and quantified using MAM approach, including oxidations of Met and Trp, glycation, cysteine variants, truncation, mutations, etc. Those PTMs

Peak	N-terminal structure of light chains	Relative content (%)
Acidic	pyroGlu/pyroGlu	5.26 ± 0.01
M	pyroGlu/pyroGlu	89.40 ± 0.12
B1	pyroGlu/pyroGlu	3.42 ± 0.08
B2	Gln/pyroGlu	1.92 ± 0.05

M: major and B: basic.

Table 8. The relative contents of N-terminal cyclization variant from rituximab identified by CEX analysis.

Peptide	Number	Change	Calculated mass (Da)	Mass (Da)	Error (ppm)	Relative content (%)
QIVLSQSPAI LSASPGEK	L:T1		1823.9993	1823.9949	−2.41	0.93 ± 0.01
pEIVLSQSPAI LSASPGEK	L:T1	pyroGlu	1806.9727	1806.9731	0.22	99.08 ± 0.01

L: light chain, T: tryptic peptide, and pE: pyro-glutamate.

Table 9. The relative contents of N-terminal cyclization variant from rituximab identified by MAM analysis.

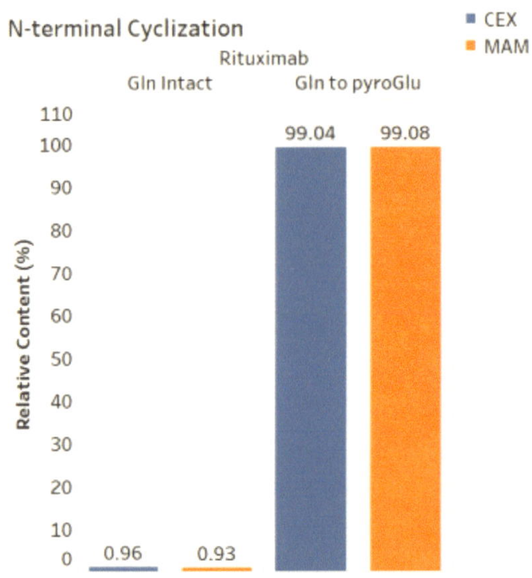

Figure 17. Profiles of N-terminal cyclization variants for rituximab.

result in mass shifts compared to those intact peptides, and this gives clues for detecting PTMs by considering the mass differences. Most of those PTMs may not be separated from their unmodified form by conventional approaches. For those cases, MAM approach is a possible alternative for quantifying those PTMs.

http://dx.doi.org/10.5772/intechopen.79107

4. Conclusions

The analytical characterization of biopharmaceutical is still challenging for biotech industry to meet the requirements. Conventional methods, such as chromatography and electrophoresis, are routinely used because they are easy to use, robust, and, cost effective. Current trends for characterization are in-depth and well characterized. Current advances in instrumentation can help to follow those trends and characterize very complex heterogeneity from various PTMs. MS is the most powerful instrument among them, which provides high resolution, accurate, and confident data with rich information from primary structure (intact mass and peptide mapping) to high order structures (PTMs and HDX).

In this chapter, several workflows are summarized for intact mass determination, primary structure analysis, and determination and quantitation of various PTMs using chromatography with online detection by MS. Those conventional approaches were assessed by the current MAM approaches primarily by peptide mapping analysis using MS.

MAM approach has been introduced, which is able to identify and quantify several attributes at once. In this chapter, glycosylation, deamidation/isomerization, C-terminal Lys variants, and N-terminal cyclization are investigated by using MAM approach, and the performance was compared to the conventional methods such as HILIC oligosaccharide analysis and CEX charge variant analysis. The results confirmed that MAM approach is quite comparable for those from conventional independent approaches.

In this chapter, we showed that MAM approach for biopharmaceutical characterization is quite comparable for typical conventional approaches using HILIC and CEX. This result conveys that MAM workflow can be extended to other related area of biopharmaceutical development as follows. MAM approach may help to select best cell lines for producing biopharmaceuticals, to support process control for upstream and downstream, and monitor critical attributes for production. MAM approach will also gain attention for the development of biosimilar requiring in-depth structural analysis for similarity.

Acknowledgements

This research was partially supported by Industry-Academy Cooperation Program of SMIT funded by BIOnSYSTEMS Ltd., Republic of Korea. Woojeong Kim was supported by the National Research Foundation of Korea (NRF) and the Center for Women In Science, Engineering and Technology (WISET) Grant funded by the Ministry of Science and ICT (MSIT) under the Program for Returners into R&D, Republic of Korea.

Conflict of interest

The authors have nothing to disclose.

Author details

Woojeong Kim[1], Kui Hyun Kang[1] and Jung-Keun Suh[2,3]*

*Address all correspondence to: jksuh@smit.ac.kr

1 BIOnSYSTEMS, Research Center, Seongnam-si, Gyeonggi-do, Republic of Korea

2 Immersive Media Lab, Seoul Media Institute of Technology, Seoul, Republic of Korea

3 Seoul Media Institute of Technology, Seoul, Republic of Korea

References

[1] Parr MK, Montacir O, Montacir H. Physicochemical characterization of biopharmaceuticals. Journal of Pharmaceutical and Biomedical Analysis. 2016;**130**:366-389. DOI: 10.1016/j.jpba.2016.05.028

[2] The MJ. Human insulin: DNA technology's first drug. American Journal of Hospital Pharmacy. 1989;**46**(11 Suppl 2):S9-S11

[3] Walsh G. Biopharmaceutical benchmarks 2014. Nature Biotechnology. 2014;**32**:992-100. DOI: 10.1038/nbt.3040

[4] Sato AK, Viswanathan M, Kent RB, Wood CR. Therapeutic peptides: Technological advances driving peptides into development. Current Opinion in Biotechnology. 2006;**17**:638-642. DOI: 10.1016/j.copbio.2006.10.002

[5] Uhlig T, Kyprianou T, Martinelli FG, Oppici CA, Heiligers D, Hills D, Calvo XR, Verhaert P. The emergence of peptides in the pharmaceuticalbusiness: From exploration to exploitation. EuPA Open Proteomics. 2014;**4**:58-69. DOI: 10.1016/j.euprot.2014.05.003

[6] Jafari R, Zolbanin NM, Rafatpanah H, Majidi J, Kazemi T. Fc-fusion proteins in therapy: An updated view. Current Medicinal Chemistry. 2017;**24**(12):1228-1237. DOI: 10.2174/0929867324666170113112759

[7] Rogstad S, Faustino A, Ruth A, Keire D, Boyne M, Park J. A retrospective evaluation of the use of mass spectrometry in FDA biologics license applications. Journal of the American Society for Mass Spectrometry. 2017;**28**:786-794. DOI: 10.1007/s13361-016-1531-9

[8] Top 20 Drugs in the World 2017 [Internet]. Available from: https://igeahub.com/2017/08/08/top-20-drugs-in-the-world-2017/ [Accessed: 01-04-2018]

[9] Zolot RS, Basu S, Million RP. Antibody-drug conjugates. Nature Reviews. Drug Discovery. 2013;**12**(4):259-260. DOI: 10.1038/nrd3980

[10] Carter PJ, Lazar GA. Next generation antibody drugs: Pursuit of the 'high-hanging fruit. Nature Reviews. Drug Discovery. 2018;**17**(3):197-223. DOI: 10.1038/nrd.2017.227

[11] Wakankar A, Chen Y, Gokarn Y, Jacobson FS. Analytical methods for physicochemical characterization of antibody drug conjugates. MAbs. 2011;**3**(2):161-172. DOI: 10.4161/mabs.3.2.14960

[12] Fan G, Wang Z, Hao M, Li J. Bispecific antibodies and their applications. Journal of Hematology & Oncology. 2015;**8**:130. DOI: 10.1186/s13045-015-0227-0

[13] De Nardis C, Hendriks LJA, Poirier E, Arvinte T, Gros P, Bakker ABH, de Kruif J. A new approach for generating bispecific antibodies based on a common light chain format and the stable architecture of human immunoglobulin G(1). The Journal of Biological Chemistry. 2017;**292**(35):14706-14717. DOI: 10.1074/jbc.M117.793497

[14] Godar M, de Haard H, Blanchetot C, Rasser J. Therapeutic bispecific antibody formats: A patent applications review (1994-2017). Expert Opinion on Therapeutic Patents. 2018;**28**(3):251-276. DOI: 10.1080/13543776.2018.1428307

[15] Strohl WR. Current progress in innovative engineered antibodies. Protein & Cell. 2018;**9**(1):86-120. DOI: 10.1007/s13238-017-0457-8

[16] Johnson JA. Biologics and Biosimilars: Background and Key Issues. CRS Report. 2017;R44620. Available from: https://fas.org/sgp/crs/misc/R44620.pdf

[17] Crespi-Lofton J, Skelton JB. The growing role of biologics and biosimilars in the United States: Perspectives from the APhA Biologics and Biosimilars Stakeholder Conference. Journal of the American Pharmaceutical Association. 2017;**57**(5):e15-e27. DOI: 10.1016/j.japh.2017.05.014

[18] Peterson J, Budlong H, Affeldt T, Skiermont K, Kyllo G, Heaton A. Biosimilar products in the modern U.S. health care and regulatory landscape. Journal of Managed Care & Specialty Pharmacy. 2017;**23**(12):1255-1259. DOI: 10.18553/jmcp.2017.23.12.1255

[19] U.S. Food and Drug Administration. Biosimilar and Interchangeable Products [Internet]. Available from: https://www.fda.gov/Drugs/DevelopmentApprovalProcess/HowDrugsareDevelopedandApproved/ApprovalApplications/TherapeuticBiologicApplications/Biosimilars/ucm580419.htm [Accessed: 15-04-2018]

[20] Song KE, Byeon J, Moon DB, Kim HH, Choi Y-J, Suh J-K. Structural identification of modified amino acids on the interface between EPO and its receptor from EPO BRP, human recombinant erythropoietin by LC/MS analysis. Molecules and Cells. 2014;**37**(11):819-826. DOI: 10.14348/molcells.2014.0214

[21] Byeon J, Choi Y-J, Suh J-K. Structural characterization of modification on the interface between a ligand and its receptor for biopharmaceuticals. Receptors & Clinical Investigation. 2015;**2**(2):1-5. DOI: 10.14800/rci.536

[22] Byeon J, Kang KH, Jung H-K, Suh J-K. Assessment for quantification of biopharmaceutical protein using a microvolume spectrometer on microfluidic slides. BioChip Journal. 2017;**11**(1):21-29. DOI: 10.1007/s13206-016-1104-9

[23] International Conference on Harmonisation of Technical Requirements for Registration of Pharmaceuticals for Human Use. ICH Q5E guideline, Comparability of biotechnological/biological products subject to changes in their manufacturing process. 2004

[24] International Conference on Harmonisation of Technical Requirements for Registration of Pharmaceuticals for Human Use. ICH Q6B guideline, Specifications: Test Procedures and Acceptance Criteria for Biotechnological/Biological Products. 1999

[25] International Conference on Harmonisation of Technical Requirements for Registration of Pharmaceuticals for Human Use. ICH Q8 R2 guideline, Pharmaceutical development. 2009. Available from: https://www.ich.org/fileadmin/Public_Web_Site/ICH_Products/Guidelines/Quality/ Q8_R1/Step4/Q8_R2_Guideline.pdf

[26] Li Y, Champion MM, Sun L, Champion PA, Wojcik R, Dovichi NJ. Capillary zone electrophoresis-electrospray ionization-tandem mass spectrometry as an alternative proteomics platform to ultraperformance liquid chromatography-electrospray ionization-tandem mass spectrometry for samples of intermediate complexity. Analytical Chemistry. 2012;**84**(3):1617-1622. DOI: 10.1021/ac202899p

[27] Srebalus Barnes CA, Lim A. Applications of mass spectrometry for the structural characterization of recombinant protein pharmaceuticals. Mass Spectrometry Reviews. 2007;**26**(3):370-388. DOI: 10.1002/mas.20129

[28] Bondarenko PV, Second TP, Zabrouskov V, Makarov AA, Zhang Z. Mass measurement and top-down HPLC/MS analysis of intact monoclonal antibodies on a hybrid linear quadrupole ion trap-Orbitrap mass spectrometer. Journal of the American Society for Mass Spectrometry. 2009;**20**(8):1415-1424. DOI: 10.1016/j.jasms.2009.03.020

[29] Tran BQ, Barton C, Feng J, Sandjong A, Yoon SH, Awasthi S, Liang T, Khan MM, Kilgour DPA, Goodlett DR, Goo YA. Comprehensive glycosylation profiling of IgG and IgG-fusion proteins by top-down MS with multiple fragmentation techniques. Journal of Proteomics. 2016;**134**:93-101. DOI: 10.1016/j.jprot.2015.10.021

[30] He L, Anderson LC, Barnidge DR, Murray DL, Hendrickson CL, Marshall AG. Analysis of monoclonal antibodies in human serum as a model for clinical monoclonal Gammopathy by use of 21 tesla FT-ICR top-down and middle-down MS/MS. Journal of the American Society for Mass Spectrometry. 2017;**28**(5):827-838. DOI: 10.1007/s13361-017-1602-6

[31] Thompson NJ, Rosati S, Heck AJ. Performing native mass spectrometry analysis on therapeutic antibodies. Methods. 2014;**65**(1):11-17. DOI: 10.1016/j.ymeth.2013.05.003

[32] Beck A, Debaene F, Diemer H, Wagner-Rousset E, Colas O, Van Dorsselaer A, Cianférani S. Cutting-edge mass spectrometry characterization of originator, biosimilar and biobetter antibodies. Journal of Mass Spectrometry. 2015;**50**(2):285-297. DOI: 10.1002/jms.3554

[33] Siuti N, Kelleher NL. Decoding protein modifications using top-down mass spectrometry. Nature Methods. 2007;**4**(10):817-821. DOI: 10.1038/nmeth1097

[34] Macht M. Top-down characterization of biopharmaceuticals. Trends in Analytical Chemistry. 2013;**48**:62-71. DOI: 10.1016/j.trac.2013.01.016

[35] Liu L. Antibody glycosylation and its impact on the pharmacokinetics and pharmacodynamics of monoclonal antibodies and Fc-fusion proteins. Journal of Pharmaceutical Sciences. 2015;**104**(6):1866-1884. DOI: 10.1002/jps.24444

[36] Zhang Z, Pan H, Chen X. Mass spectrometry for structural characterization of therapeutic antibodies. Mass Spectrometry Reviews. 2009;**28**(1):147-176. DOI: 10.1002/mas.20190

[37] Ayoub D, Jabs W, Resemann A, Evers W, Evans C, Main L, Baessmann C, Wagner-Rousset E, Suckau D, Beck A. Correct primary structure assessment and extensive glyco-profiling of cetuximab by a combination of intact, middle-up, middle-down and bottom-up ESI and MALDI mass spectrometry techniques. MAbs. 2013;**5**(5):699-710. DOI: 10.4161/mabs.25423

[38] Wang B, Gucinski AC, Keire DA, Buhse LF, Boyne MT 2nd. Structural comparison of two anti-CD20 monoclonal antibody drug products using middle-down mass spectrometry. The Analyst. 2013;**138**(10):3058-3065. DOI: 10.1039/c3an36524g

[39] Fornelli L, Ayoub D, Aizikov K, Beck A, Tsybin YO. Middle-down analysis of monoclonal antibodies with electron transfer dissociation orbitrap fourier transform mass spectrometry. Analytical Chemistry. 2014;**86**(6):3005-3012. DOI: 10.1021/ac4036857

[40] Hartman PA, Stodola JD, Harbour GC, Hoogerheide JG. Reversed-phase high-performance liquid chromatography peptide mapping of bovine somatotropin. Journal of Chromatography. 1986;**360**(2):385-395. DOI: 10.1016/S0021-9673(00)91687-X

[41] Recny MA, Scoble HA, Kim Y. Structural characterization of natural human urinary and recombinant DNA-derived erythropoietin. Identification of des-arginine 166 erythropoietin. The Journal of Biological Chemistry. 1987;**262**(35):17156-17163. Available from: http://www.jbc.org/content/262/35/17156.full.pdf

[42] Dougherty JJ Jr, Snyder LM, Sinclair RL, Robins RH. High-performance tryptic mapping of recombinant bovine somatotropin. Analytical Biochemistry. 1990;**190**(1):7-20. DOI: 10.1016/0003-2697(90)90126-T

[43] Schär M, Börnsen KO, Gassmann E. Fast protein sequence determination with matrix-assisted laser desorption and ionization mass spectrometry. Rapid Communications in Mass Spectrometry. 1991;**5**(7):319-326. DOI: 10.1002/rcm.1290050705

[44] Bongers J, Cummings JJ, Ebert MB, Federici MM, Gledhill L, Gulati D, Hilliard GM, Jones BH, Lee KR, Mozdzanowski J, Naimoli M, Burman S. Validation of a peptide mapping method for a therapeutic monoclonal antibody: What could we possibly learn about a method we have run 100 times? Journal of Pharmaceutical and Biomedical Analysis. 2000;**21**(6):1099-1128. DOI: 10.1016/S0731-7085(99)00181-8

[45] Hernandez P, Müller M, Appel RD. Automated protein identification by tandem mass spectrometry: Issues and strategies. Mass Spectrometry Reviews. 2006;**25**(2):235-254. DOI: 10.1002/mas.20068

[46] Zhang Y, Fonslow BR, Shan B, Baek MC, Yates JR 3rd. Protein analysis by shotgun/bottom-up proteomics. Chemical Reviews. 2013;**113**(4):2343-2494. DOI: 10.1021/cr3003533

[47] Byeon J, Yim Y-R, Kim H-H, Suh J-K. Structural identification of a non-glycosylated variant at Ser126 for O-glycosylation site from EPO BRP, human recombinant erythropoietin by LC/MS analysis. Molecules and Cells. 2015;**38**(6):496-505. DOI: 10.14348/molcells.2015.2256

[48] Wang Y, Li X, Liu YH, Richardson D, Li H, Shameem M, Yang X. Simultaneous monitoring of oxidation, deamidation, isomerization, and glycosylation of monoclonal antibodies by liquid chromatography-mass spectrometry method with ultrafast tryptic digestion. MAbs. 2016;**8**(8):1477-1486. DOI: 10.1080/19420862.2016.1226715

[49] Pace CN, Vajdos F, Fee L, Grimsley G, Gray T. How to measure and predict the molar absorption coefficient of a protein. Protein Science. 1995;**4**(11):2411-2423. DOI: 10.1002/pro.5560041120

[50] Proc JL, Kuzyk MA, Hardie DB, Yang J, Smith DS, Jackson AM, Parker CE, Borchers CH. A quantitative study of the effects of chaotropic agents, surfactants, and solvents on the digestion efficiency of human plasma proteins by trypsin. Journal of Proteome Research. 2010;**9**(10):5422-5437. DOI: 10.1021/pr100656u

[51] Yu YQ, Gilar M, Lee PJ, Bouvier ES, Gebler JC. Enzyme-friendly, mass spectrometry-compatible surfactant for in-solution enzymatic digestion of proteins. Analytical Chemistry. 2003;**75**(21):6023-6028. DOI: 10.1021/ac0346196

[52] Han JC, Han GY. A procedure for quantitative determination of tris(2-carboxyethyl) phosphine, an odorless reducing agent more stable and effective than dithiothreitol. Analytical Biochemistry. 1994;**220**(1):5-10. DOI: 10.1006/abio.1994.1290

[53] Svoboda M, Meister W, Vetter W. A method for counting disulfide bridges in small proteins by reduction with mercaptoethanol and electrospray mass spectrometry. Journal of Mass Spectrometry. 1995;**30**:1562-1566. DOI: 10.1002/jms.1190301107

[54] Switzar L, Giera M, Niessen WM. Protein digestion: An overview of the available techniques and recent developments. Journal of Proteome Research. 2013;**12**(3):1067-1077. DOI: 10.1021/pr301201x

[55] Tsiatsiani L, Heck AJ. Proteomics beyond trypsin. The FEBS Journal. 2015;**282**(14):2612-2626. DOI: 10.1111/febs.13287

[56] Bunkenborg J, Espadas G, Molina H. Cutting edge proteomics: Benchmarking of six commercial trypsins. Journal of Proteome Research. 2013;**12**(8):3631-3641. DOI: 10.1021/pr4001465

[57] Giansanti P, Tsiatsiani L, Low TY, Heck AJ. Six alternative proteases for mass spectrometry-based proteomics beyond trypsin. Nature Protocols. 2016;**11**(5):993-1006. DOI: 10.1038/nprot.2016.057

[58] Plumb R, Castro-Perez J, Granger J, Beattie I, Joncour K, Wright A. Ultra-performance liquid chromatography coupled to quadrupole-orthogonal time-of-flight mass spectrometry. Rapid Communications in Mass Spectrometry. 2004;**18**(19):2331-2337. DOI: 10.1002/rcm.1627

[59] Motoyama A, Venable JD, Ruse CI, Yates JR 3rd. Automated ultra-high-pressure multidimensional protein identification technology (UHP-MudPIT) for improved peptide identification of proteomic samples. Analytical Chemistry. 2006;**78**(14):5109-5118. DOI: 10.1021/ac060354u

[60] Omamogho JO, Glennon JD. Comparison between the efficiencies of sub-2 μm C18 particles packed in narrow bore columns. Analytical Chemistry. 2011;**83**(5):1547-1556. DOI: 10.1021/ac102139a

[61] Water TH. Recent innovations in UHPLC columns and instrumentation. Trends in Analytical Chemistry. 2014;**63**:14-20. DOI: 10.1016/j.trac.2014.07.016

[62] González-Ruiz V, Olives AI, Martín MA. Core-shell particles lead the way to renewing high-performance liquid chromatography. Trends in Analytical Chemistry. 2015;**64**:17-28. DOI: 10.1016/j.trac.2014.08.008

[63] Kochling J, Wu W, Hua Y, Guan Q, Castaneda-Merced J. A platform analytical quality by design (AQbD) approach for multiple UHPLC-UV and UHPLC-MS methods development for protein analysis. Journal of Pharmaceutical and Biomedical Analysis. 2016;**125**:130-139. DOI: 10.1016/j.jpba.2016.03.031

[64] Ghosh PK. Introduction to Protein Mass Spectrometry. 1st ed. London: Academic Press; 2015. Available from: https://www.sciencedirect.com/science/book/9780128021026

[65] Domon B, Aebersold R. Mass spectrometry and protein analysis. Science. 2006;**312**(5771): 212-217. DOI: 10.1126/science.1124619

[66] Yu L, Remmele RL Jr, He B. Identification of N-terminal modification for recombinant monoclonal antibody light chain using partial reduction and quadrupole time-of-flight mass spectrometry. Rapid Communications in Mass Spectrometry. 2006;**20**(24):3674-3680. DOI: 10.1002/rcm.2790

[67] Wang D, Wynne C, Gu F, Becker C, Zhao J, Mueller HM, Li H, Shameem M, Liu YH. Characterization of drug-product-related impurities and variants of a therapeutic monoclonal antibody by higher energy C-trap dissociation mass spectrometry. Analytical Chemistry. 2015;**87**(2):914-921. DOI: 10.1021/ac503158g

[68] Colgrave ML, Craik DJ. Thermal, chemical, and enzymatic stability of the cyclotide kalata B1: The importance of the cyclic cystine knot. Biochemistry. 2004;**43**(20):5965-5975. DOI: 10.1021/bi049711q

[69] Fass D. Disulfide bonding in protein biophysics. Annual Review of Biophysics. 2012;**41**: 63-79. DOI: 10.1146/annurev-biophys-050511-102321

[70] Goyder MS, Rebeaud F, Pfeifer ME, Kálmán F. Strategies in mass spectrometry for the assignment of Cys-Cys disulfide connectivities in proteins. Expert Review of Proteomics. 2013;**10**(5):489-501. DOI: 10.1586/14789450.2013.837663

[71] Wiesner J, Resemann A, Evans C, Suckau D, Jabs W. Advanced mass spectrometry workflows for analyzing disulfide bonds in biologics. Expert Review of Proteomics. 2015;**12**(2):115-123. DOI: 10.1586/14789450.2015.1018896

[72] Gorman JJ, Wallis TP, Pitt JJ. Protein disulfide bond determination by mass spectrometry. Mass Spectrometry Reviews. 2002;**21**(3):183-216. DOI: 10.1002/mas.10025

[73] Lakbub JC, Shipman JT, Desaire H. Recent mass spectrometry-based techniques and considerations for disulfide bond characterization in proteins. Analytical and Bioanalytical Chemistry. 2018;**410**(10):2467-2484. DOI: 10.1007/s00216-017-0772-1

[74] Liu H, May K. Disulfide bond structures of IgG molecules: Structural variations, chemical modifications and possible impacts to stability and biological function. MAbs. 2012;**4**(1):17-23. DOI: 10.4161/mabs.4.1.18347

[75] Wu SL, Jiang H, Hancock WS, Karger BL. Identification of the unpaired cysteine status and complete mapping of the 17 disulfides of recombinant tissue plasminogen activator using LC-MS with electron transfer dissociation/collision induced dissociation. Analytical Chemistry. 2010;**82**(12):5296-5303. DOI: 10.1021/ac100766r

[76] Wu SL, Jiang H, Lu Q, Dai S, Hancock WS, Karger BL. Mass spectrometric determination of disulfide linkages in recombinant therapeutic proteins using online LC-MS with electron-transfer dissociation. Analytical Chemistry. 2009;**81**(1):112-122. DOI: 10.1021/ac801560k

[77] Xie H, Gilar M, Gebler JC. Characterization of protein impurities and site-specific modifications using peptide mapping with liquid chromatography and data independent acquisition mass spectrometry. Analytical Chemistry. 2009;**81**(14):5699-5708. DOI: 10.1021/ac900468j

[78] Xie H, Chakraborty AB, Chen W. Towards fast mapping of protein disulfide bonds: An integrated workflow for automatic assignment of disulfide pairing. In: Proceedings of Practical Applications of Mass Spectrometry in the Biotechnology Industry; 8-10 September 2010; Marina Del Ray. CA: Mass Spec; 2010. p. 107. Available from: http://www.waters.com/webassets/cms/ library/docs/720003751en.pdf

[79] Walsh CT, Garneau-Tsodikova S, Gatto GJ Jr. Protein posttranslational modifications: The chemistry of proteome diversifications. Angewandte Chemie (International Ed. in English). 2005;**44**(45):7342-7372. DOI: 10.1002/anie.200501023

[80] Li W, Kerwin JL, Schiel J, Formolo T, Davis D, Mahan A, Benchaar SA. Structural elucidation of post-translational modifications in monoclonal antibodies. In: Schiel JE, Davis DL, Borisov OV, editors. State-of-the-art and Emerging Technologies for Therapeutic Monoclonal Antibody Characterization Volume 2. Biopharmaceutical Characterization: The NIST mAb Case Study. Washington, DC: American Chemical Society; 2015. pp. 119-183. DOI: 10.1021/bk-2015-1201.ch003

[81] Walsh G. Post-translational modifications of protein biopharmaceuticals. Drug Discovery Today. 2010;**15**:773-780. DOI: 10.1016/j.drudis.2010.06.009

[82] Brinks V, Hawe A, Basmeleh AH, Joachin-Rodriguez L, Haselberg R, Somsen GW, Jis5oot W, Schellekens H. Quality of original and biosimilar epoetin products. Pharmaceutical Research. 2011;**28**(2):386-393. DOI: 10.1007/s11095-010-0288-2

[83] Berkowitz SA, Engen JR, Mazzeo JR, Jones GB. Analytical tools for characterizing biopharmaceuticals and the implications for biosimilars. Nature Reviews. Drug Discovery. 2012;**11**:527-540. DOI: 10.1038/nrd3746

[84] Diepold K, Bomans K, Wiedmann M, Zimmermann B, Petzold A, Schlothauer T, Mueller R, Moritz B, Stracke JO, Mølhøj M, Reusch D, Bulau P. Simultaneous assessment of Asp isomerization and Asn deamidation in recombinant antibodies by LC-MS following incubation at elevated temperatures. PLoS One. 2012;**7**(1):e30295. DOI: 10.1371/journal.pone.0030295

[85] Beck A, Wagner-Rousset E, Ayoub D, Van Dorsselaer A, Sanglier-Cianferani S. Characterization of therapeutic antibodies and related products. Analytical Chemistry. 2013;**85**:715-736. DOI: 10.1021/ac3032355

[86] Fekete S, Guillarme D, Sandra P, Sandra K. Chromatographic, electrophoretic, and mass spectrometric methods for the analytical characterization of protein biopharmaceuticals. Analytical Chemistry. 2016;**88**:480-507. DOI: 10.1021/acs.analchem.5b04561

[87] Rogers RS, Nightlinger NS, Livingston B, Campbell P, Bailey R, Balland A. Development of a quantitative mass spectrometry multiattribute method for characterization, quality control testing and disposition of biologics. MAbs. 2015;**7**:881-890. DOI: 10.1080/19420862

[88] Wang T, Chu L, Li W, Lawson K, Apostol I, Eris T. Application of a quantitative LC–MS multiattribute method for monitoring site-specific glycan heterogeneity on a monoclonal antibody containing two N-linked glycosylation sites. Analytical Chemistry. 2017;**89**:3562-3567. DOI: 10.1021/acs.analchem.6b04856

[89] Huhn C, Selman MH, Ruhaak LR, Deelder AM, Wuhrer M. IgG glycosylation analysis. Proteomics. 2009;**9**(4):882-913. DOI: 10.1002/pmic.200800715

[90] Abès R, Teillaud JL. Impact of glycosylation on effector functions of therapeutic IgG. Pharmaceuticals (Basel). 2010;**3**(1):146-157. DOI: 10.3390/ph3010146

[91] Sibéril S, Dutertre CA, Fridman WH, Teillaud JL, Fcgamma R. The key to optimize therapeutic antibodies? Critical Reviews in Oncology/Hematology. 2007;**62**(1):26-33. DOI: 10.1016/j.critrevonc.2006.12.003

[92] Takahashi M, Kuroki Y, Ohtsubo K, Taniguchi N. Core fucose and bisecting GlcNAc, the direct modifiers of the N-glycan core: Their functions and target proteins. Carbohydrate Research. 2009;**344**(12):1387-1390. DOI: 10.1016/j.carres.2009.04.031

[93] Abès R, Dutertre CA, Agnelli L, Teillaud JL. Activating and inhibitory Fcgamma receptors in immunotherapy: Being the actor or being the target. Expert Review of Clinical Immunology. 2009;**5**(6):735-747. DOI: 10.1586/eci.09.57

[94] Zhang Q, Li Z, Wang Y, Zheng Q, Li J. Mass spectrometry for protein sialoglycosylation. Mass Spectrometry Reviews. 2017. DOI: 10.1002/mas.21555

[95] Tharmalingam T, Adamczyk B, Doherty MA, Royle L, Rudd PM. Strategies for the profiling, characterisation and detailed structural analysis of N-linked oligosaccharides. Glycoconjugate Journal. 2013;**30**(2):137-146. DOI: 10.1007/s10719-012-9443-9

[96] Lauber MA, Yu YQ, Brousmiche DW, Hua Z, Koza SM, Magnelli P, Guthrie E, Taron CH, Fountain KJ. Rapid preparation of released N-glycans for HILIC analysis using a labeling reagent that facilitates sensitive fluorescence and ESI-MS detection. Analytical Chemistry. 2015;**87**(10):5401-5409. DOI: 10.1021/acs.analchem.5b00758

[97] Reusch D, Haberger M, Falck D, Peter B, Maier B, Gassner J, Hook M, Wagner K, Bonnington L, Bulau P, Wuhrer M. Comparison of methods for the analysis of therapeutic immunoglobulin G Fc-glycosylation profiles-part 2: Mass spectrometric methods. MAbs. 2015;**7**(4):732-742. DOI: 10.1080/19420862.2015.1045173

[98] Terashima I, Koga A, Nagai H. Identification of deamidation and isomerization sites on pharmaceutical recombinant antibody using H(2)(18)O. Analytical Biochemistry. 2007;**368**(1):49-60. DOI: 10.1016/j.ab.2007.05.012

[99] Liu H, Gaza-Bulseco G, Chumsae C. Glutamine deamidation of a recombinant monoclonal antibody. Rapid Communications in Mass Spectrometry. 2008;**22**(24):4081-4088. DOI: 10.1002/rcm.3831

[100] Yang H, Zubarev RA. Mass spectrometric analysis of asparagine deamidation and aspartate isomerization in polypeptides. Electrophoresis. 2010;**31**(11):1764-1772. DOI: 10.1002/elps.201000027

[101] Robinson AB, Scotchler JW, McKerrow JH. Rates of nonenzymatic deamidation of glutaminyl and asparaginyl residues in pentapeptides. Journal of the American Chemical Society. 1973;**95**(24):8156-8159

[102] Scotchler JW, Robinson AB. Deamidation of glutaminyl residues: Dependence on pH, temperature, and ionic strength. Analytical Biochemistry. 1974;**59**(1):319-322. DOI: 10.1016/0003-2697(74)90040-2

[103] Tyler-Cross R, Schirch V. Effects of amino acid sequence, buffers, and ionic strength on the rate and mechanism of deamidation of asparagine residues in small peptides. The Journal of Biological Chemistry. 1991 Nov 25;**266**(33):22549-22556. Available from: http://www.jbc.org/content/266/33/22549.full.pdf

[104] Geiger T, Clarke S. Deamidation, isomerization, and racemization at asparaginyl and aspartyl residues in peptides. Succinimide-linked reactions that contribute to protein degradation. The Journal of Biological Chemistry. 1987;**262**(2):785-794. Available from: http://www.jbc.org/content/262/2/785.full.pdf

[105] Wakankar AA, Borchardt RT, Eigenbrot C, Shia S, Wang YJ, Shire SJ, Liu JL. Aspartate isomerization in the complementarity-determining regions of two closely related monoclonal antibodies. Biochemistry. 2007;**46**(6):1534-1544. DOI: 10.1021/bi061500t

[106] Sreedhara A, Cordoba A, Zhu Q, Kwong J, Liu J. Characterization of the isomerization products of aspartate residues at two different sites in a monoclonal antibody. Pharmaceutical Research. 2012;**29**(1):187-197. DOI: 10.1007/s11095-011-0534-2

[107] Liu H, Gaza-Bulseco G, Faldu D, Chumsae C, Sun J. Heterogeneity of monoclonal antibodies. Journal of Pharmaceutical Sciences. 2008;**97**(7):2426-2447. DOI: 10.1002/jps.21180

[108] Wakankar AA, Liu J, Vandervelde D, Wang YJ, Shire SJ, Borchardt RT. The effect of cosolutes on the isomerization of aspartic acid residues and conformational stability in a monoclonal antibody. Journal of Pharmaceutical Sciences. 2007;**96**(7):1708-1718. DOI: 10.1002/jps.20823

[109] Rehder DS, Chelius D, McAuley A, Dillon TM, Xiao G, Crouse-Zeineddini J, Vardanyan L, Perico N, Mukku V, Brems DN, Matsumura M, Bondarenko PV. Isomerization of a single aspartyl residue of anti-epidermal growth factor receptor immunoglobulin gamma2 antibody highlights the role avidity plays in antibody activity. Biochemistry. 2008;**47**(8):2518-2530. DOI: 10.1021/bi7018223

[110] Yan Y, Wei H, Fu Y, Jusuf S, Zeng M, Ludwig R, Krystek SR Jr, Chen G, Tao L, Das TK. Isomerization and oxidation in the complementarity-determining regions of a monoclonal antibody: A study of the modification-structure-function correlations by hydrogen-deuterium exchange mass spectrometry. Analytical Chemistry. 2016;**88**(4):2041-2050. DOI: 10.1021/acs.analchem.5b02800

[111] Harris RJ, Kabakoff B, Macchi FD, Shen FJ, Kwong M, Andya JD, Shire SJ, Bjork N, Totpal K, Chen AB. Identification of multiple sources of charge heterogeneity in a recombinant antibody. Journal of Chromatography. B, Biomedical Sciences and Applications. 2001;**752**(2):233-245. DOI: 10.1016/S0378-4347(00)00548-X

[112] Chu GC, Chelius D, Xiao G, Khor HK, Coulibaly S, Bondarenko PV. Accumulation of succinimide in a recombinant monoclonal antibody in mildly acidic buffers under elevated temperatures. Pharmaceutical Research. 2007;**24**(6):1145-1156. DOI: 10.1007/s11095-007-9241-4

[113] Kroon DJ, Baldwin-Ferro A, Lalan P. Identification of sites of degradation in a therapeutic monoclonal antibody by peptide mapping. Pharmaceutical Research. 1992;**9**(11):1386-1393

[114] Chelius D, Rehder DS, Bondarenko PV. Identification and characterization of deamidation sites in the conserved regions of human immunoglobulin gamma antibodies. Analytical Chemistry. 2005;**77**(18):6004-6011. DOI: 10.1021/ac050672d

[115] Dick LW Jr, Qiu D, Mahon D, Adamo M, Cheng KC. C-terminal lysine variants in fully human monoclonal antibodies: Investigation of test methods and possible causes. Biotechnology and Bioengineering. 2008;**100**(6):1132-1143. DOI: 10.1002/bit.21855

[116] Luo J, Zhang J, Ren D, Tsai WL, Li F, Amanullah A, Hudson T. Probing of C-terminal lysine variation in a recombinant monoclonal antibody production using Chinese hamster ovary cells with chemically defined media. Biotechnology and Bioengineering. 2012;**109**(9):2306-2315. DOI: 10.1002/bit.24510

[117] Jiang G, Yu C, Yadav DB, Hu Z, Amurao A, Duenas E, Wong M, Iverson M, Zheng K, Lam X, Chen J, Vega R, Ulufatu S, Leddy C, Davis H, Shen A, Wong PY, Harris R, Wang YJ, Li D. Evaluation of heavy-chain C-terminal deletion on product quality and pharmacokinetics of monoclonal antibodies. Journal of Pharmaceutical Sciences. 2016;**105**(7):2066-2072. DOI: 10.1016/j.xphs.2016.04.027

[118] Antes B, Amon S, Rizzi A, Wiederkum S, Kainer M, Szolar O, Fido M, Kircheis R, Nechansky A. Analysis of lysine clipping of a humanized Lewis-Y specific IgG antibody and its relation to Fc-mediated effector function. Journal of Chromatography. B, Analytical Technologies in the Biomedical and Life Sciences. 2007;**852**(1-2):250-256. DOI: 10.1016/j.jchromb.2007.01.024

[119] van den Bremer ET, Beurskens FJ, Voorhorst M, Engelberts PJ, de Jong RN, van der Boom BG, Cook EM, Lindorfer MA, Taylor RP, van Berkel PH, Parren PW. Human IgG is produced in a pro-form that requires clipping of C-terminal lysines for maximal complement activation. MAbs. 2015;**7**(4):672-680. DOI: 10.1080/19420862.2015.1046665

[120] Kim DG, Kim HJ, Kim HJ. Effects of carboxypeptidase B treatment and elevated temperature on recombinant monoclonal antibody charge variants in cation-exchange chromatography analysis. Archives of Pharmacal Research. 2016;**39**(10):1472-1481. DOI: 10.1007/s12272-016-0818-5

[121] Liu J, Eris T, Li C, Cao S, Kuhns S. Assessing analytical similarity of proposed amgen biosimilar ABP 501 to adalimumab. BioDrugs. 2016;**30**(4):321-338. DOI: 10.1007/s40259-016-0184-3

[122] Miao S, Fan L, Zhao L, Ding D, Liu X, Wang H, Tan WS. Physicochemical and biological characterization of the proposed biosimilar tocilizumab. BioMed Research International. 2017;**2017**. DOI: 4926168. DOI: 10.1155/2017/4926168

[123] Dick LW Jr, Kim C, Qiu D, Cheng KC. Determination of the origin of the N-terminal pyroglutamate variation in monoclonal antibodies using model peptides. Biotechnology and Bioengineering. 2007;**97**(3):544-553. DOI: 10.1002/bit.21260

[124] Liu YD, Goetze AM, Bass RB, Flynn GC. N-terminal glutamate to pyroglutamate conversion in vivo for human IgG2 antibodies. The Journal of Biological Chemistry. 2011;**286**(13):11211-11217. DOI: 10.1074/jbc.M110.185041

Section 3

Development

Chapter 3

"Cell-Free Therapeutics" from Components Secreted by Mesenchymal Stromal Cells as a Novel Class of Biopharmaceuticals

Georgy D. Sagaradze, Peter P. Nimiritsky, Zhanna A. Akopyan, Pavel I. Makarevich and Anastasia Yu. Efimenko

Additional information is available at the end of the chapter

http://dx.doi.org/10.5772/intechopen.78605

Abstract

Regenerative medicine is a fast growing multidisciplinary field aiming at the regeneration or replacement of damaged cells, tissues, or organs. Adult multipotent mesenchymal stromal cells (MSCs) are often used as a principal therapeutic tool in this field. Along with differentiation potency, MSCs secrete a wide spectrum of paracrine factors and extracellular vesicles participating in tissue repair and regeneration. Thus, for injuries that require trophic stimulation, cell survival support, and/or resident stem cells activation to be restored, one can apply MSC-conditioned medium, a combination of products and extracellular vesicles in cell culture growth medium, secreted by MSC. It could mediate most of beneficial regenerative effects of MSC without possible side effects of using MSC themselves. However, before the clinical application of this promising biopharmaceutical, several issues such as manufacturing protocols, quality control, and others must be addressed. Subsequently, we highlight the questions considering donor material variability, manufacturing, cell culture medium and auxiliary components selection, and potency tests development.

Keywords: biopharmaceuticals, multipotent mesenchymal stromal cells, conditioned medium, quality control, regenerative medicine

1. Introduction

Regenerative medicine is a fast growing multidisciplinary field aiming at the regeneration or replacement of damaged cells, tissues, or organs. Adult stem and progenitor cells represent a pivotal tool in regenerative medicine. It is important to highlight mesenchymal stromal cells (MSCs) as the most popular source for cell therapy and tissue engineering. However, a large amount of experimental data indicate that MSC effects on regeneration are mostly mediated by their ability to produce a wide range of bioactive molecules, and the use of MSC-conditioned medium (CM), a complex of the factors secreted to cell culture growth medium, as a distinct biopharmaceutical drug can be a rational alternative to direct MSC therapy. MSC CM could be considered as "cell-free therapeutics" since this product is devoid of MSC themselves in its final formulation, yet possess significant therapeutic potency. It contains components secreted by MSC and reproduced the effects of MSC-based cell therapy.

"Cell-free therapeutics" have various advantages in overcoming the limitations and risks associated with the cell-based therapy. Despite the outstanding preclinical and clinical efficacy of MSC CM, there is still no generally accepted regulating approaches for CM standardization and quality control. This chapter reviews the current state of art in the development of MSC CM-based medicinal products and describes the crucial issues concerning the production and quality control of this promising class of biopharmaceuticals.

2. Physiological activity of MSC

Postnatal stem and progenitor cells are responsible for tissue renewal and regeneration throughout the whole human lifetime. Accumulating evidence indicates that stem cells function only within a specific niche. Stem cell niche is considered as a local tissue microenvironment that maintains stem cells and regulates their function by producing factors that act directly on stem cells [1]. This microenvironment provides structural cues and paracrine signals to support stemness. Mesenchymal stromal cells (MSCs) are found in many niches of tissue-specific resident stem cells. The function of MSC in a niche is often critical for its maintenance. MSC plays an important role in coupling information from the environment with stem cell populations. MSCs react to endocrine and nervous system signals: thus, the stimulation of a specific type of MSC by granulocyte colony-stimulating factor (G-CSF) or beta-3-adrenoreceptor agonists decreases the expression of the panel of genes supporting hematopoietic stem cells (HSCs). Furthermore, upon MSC, withdrawal in niche HSC activity and quantity decrease [2]. MSCs also interact with stem cells and other internal components of the niche for effective control over HSC, ensuring they support hematopoiesis without inducing aberrant proliferation. It should be noted that the maintenance of stem cells in the niche is not the only function of MSC. These cells are also involved in the formation and maintenance of a structural component of the niche. MSC isolated from a subendothelial layer of bone marrow stroma can form a microenvironment alike a miniature bone organ, similar to the HSC niche, under heterotopic transplantation. The establishment of subendothelial stromal cells in developing heterotopic BM in vivo occurs via specific, dynamic interactions with developing sinusoids. Subendothelial stromal cells are major producers of angiopoietin-1 (Angpt-1), the principal factor of HSC niche involved in vascular remodeling [3].

MSCs provide their supporting functions through secretory activity in physiological conditions. MSCs secrete a number of factors that are critical for the maintenance of stem cells in their niches [4, 5]. Consistent with other reports, we have shown that the largest functional cluster in MSC secretome is composed of extracellular matrix (ECM) proteins [6]. Such protein profile is in line with the stromal characteristics of adipose MSC. Adequate production of ECM components is necessary for tissue homeostasis and regeneration, because these molecules not only provide a scaffold for cells and soluble molecules but also regulate angiogenesis, neurogenesis, and inflammation. In addition, a large amount of data indicates that apart from soluble factors MSCs secrete regulatory non-coding RNA (e.g., micro RNA) within extracellular vesicles (EVs). The release of these small RNA by MSC can play a role in stem cell niche maintenance by controlling and tuning proliferation, differentiation, and homing. Particularly, microRNA regulates diverse biological processes, including growth and differentiation of stem cells [7, 8].

The function of adult stem cells includes the local or remote replacement of senescent or damaged cells along with maintaining their own pool. Stem cells supported by other niche components can participate in the repair of small lesions of a skin, liver, intestines, kidney, and bone marrow. However, stem cells could not cope with more serious injuries without more substantial support [9]. MSCs are important for maintaining the niche of stem cells; therefore, they can participate in stem cell potentiation to respond to damage, stimulate the survival of stem cells, and, thereby, maintain the structural and functional integrity of the niche. For example, in such serious damage as myocardium ischemia/reperfusion injury, MSC mediated its cardioprotective paracrine effect by secreting exosomes which reduced infarct size in a mouse model [10]. As in majority of animal models and clinical studies, only limited or no engraftment at all was often observed, one should consider paracrine MSC function as principal effector for tissue regeneration after, at least, systemic MSC injection for different injuries [11].

3. Rationale for use of MSC and their cell-free derivatives in regenerative medicine

MSCs are the most commonly used cells for cell-based therapy as they do not form teratomas, confer low immunogenicity, and are free of strict ethical concerns [12]. Despite these reasons, the difficulty to trace cell fate and survival in recipient has been a significant obstacle for understanding the mechanisms of the clinical efficacy that can be variable [13]. Furthermore, MSCs are highly heterogeneous and cannot be fully characterized in the context of identity and, finally, potency. At the same time, MSC CM was shown to mediate most of MSC beneficial effects. MSC CM includes various components such as cytokines, growth factors, ECM proteins and factors involved in ECM remodeling, different types of EV, and others. Using cell-free products based on biologically active factors secreted by stem and progenitor cells allows to significantly reduce the risks associated with a direct cell injection, while maintaining efficacy under wide manufacturing scalability and modification potential like fractionation, concentration, and combination with various carriers [14]. Therefore, the application of "cell-free therapeutics" based on the components secreted by MSC as a novel class of biopharmaceuticals represents a rapidly developing and promising approach in regenerative medicine.

4. Harnessing cell-free therapeutics' variability to improve their safety and efficacy

4.1. Age-related variability of MSC properties

Since MSCs are used as a starting material for CM manufacturing, it is necessary to pay attention to the standardization of MSC. The effects of this biopharmaceutical are multifactorial, and even the minimal variability of its composition can strongly affect its activity. As properties of MSC influence CM composition crucially, the variability of MSC donor characteristics and manipulations during manufacturing should be taken into account.

One of the key factors affecting MSC CM composition and therapeutic effects is a donor's age. It is generally accepted that stem cell number and/or function decline with advanced age during the replacement and the turnover of damaged cells in compromised renewable tissues. Several studies showed that MSCs derived from old donors exhibit reduced proliferative capacity, differentiation potential, and, most importantly, impaired specific activity [15]. Older adipose-derived MSC showed impaired angiogenic properties in vitro and in vivo. The production of key pro-angiogenic factors, such as vascular endothelial growth factor (VEGF), hepatocyte growth factor (HGF), and others by adipose-derived MSC, decreased with age [16]. It is important to note that factors involved in ECM remodeling like urokinase and its receptor, plasminogen activator inhibitor-1 (PAI-1), metalloproteinases 2 and 9 were overexpressed in adipose MSC from aged donors compared to younger ones, both in human and in mice [16, 17].

Furthermore, it was shown that age and age-associated conditions such as type 2 diabetes and atherosclerosis decrease the immunomodulatory capacity of human MSCs. MSCs from elderly subjects with atherosclerosis have impaired T-cell suppression compared to their non-elderly adult counterparts. Possibly, the coexistence of age and these age-related conditions could compromise MSC immunomodulatory function [18] and influence MSC CM functional properties.

Bioinformatic data also suggest that age-related changes in MSCs result in impaired therapeutic potential of aged progenitor cells [19]. In one of the studies among the most highly differentially expressed genes, transforming growth factor alpha (TGFα) overexpression in MSC from young donors was detected. TGFα has been shown to mediate the secretion of vascular endothelial growth factor A (VEGFA) by MSC, positively contributing to processes like wound healing and injury response [20]. Some other differentially expressed genes participate in MSC differentiation. As it is revealed that during early MSC differentiation, secretome of MSC can be changed, one should take into account age-related differentiation predisposition.

4.2. Sex-related variation of MSC paracrine activity

In an attempt to overcome MSC donor variation, one can explore donor sex variability. Analysis of human BM-MSC preparations to identify statistically robust influence of donor sex on MSC functional properties identified minor differences among MSC isolated from both the sexes. It was shown that high-clonogenic BM-MSCs divided more rapidly and were more frequent in BM-MSC preparations from female donors. What is more important, no correlation of donor age to adipogenic, osteogenic, and chondrogenic differentiation in vitro as confirmed by an extended panel of lineage specific markers was found. In addition, the secretion rate of molecules important for tissue regeneration and immunomodulation was analyzed. The evidence of a critical role of factors such as VEGF, platelet-derived growth factor (PDGF), hepatocyte growth factor (HGF), fibroblast growth factor 2 (FGF2), and angiopoietin-1 (Angpt-1) in contribution to male and female MSC variability was lacking [21]. As MSC-secreted factors are principal active components of MSC CM, donor sex might not influence MSC CM efficacy substantially. However, in vitro data concerning the impact of donor sex to variability of donor-derived MSC effects are controversial [22].

4.3. Variability determined by the origin of starting material for MSC isolation

MSC isolated from the most common sources can fit minimal characteristic criteria and share majority of biological properties. However, some studies demonstrated that MSCs from the popular sources such as adipose tissue and bone marrow have different transcription profiles. Among differentially expressing or expressing by only one cell type, one can find components involved in cellular communication and differentiation. Therefore, the secretory profile of different MSC types also varies. In addition, not only a spectrum of secreted paracrine factors differs but also nucleic acid, particularly microRNA composition, which might influence EV contents. The variability between EV of two types of MSC suggests that prior tissue-specific microenvironment might influence the exosomal sorting of micro-RNA. It is important as micro-RNA transferred via exosomes might be functional in repressing their targets in vitro and in vivo if transferred in high amounts [7, 23].

Taken together a plethora of donor-associated factors can influence MSC CM composition and effects. Thus to enhance the effect of this biopharmaceutical and harness lot-to-lot variability one can isolate MSC from selected donors that are optimal for MSC CM manufacturing for certain pathology.

4.4. Variability determined by manufacture process

Manufacturing features can also substantially affect the safety and efficacy of MSC CM. Among them, one can name at least optimal cell isolation protocol, growth medium selection, and cell expansion approach as well as the use of proper raw materials.

Although isolated by the same way, MSCs often demonstrate different properties when cultured in different media. The choice of medium determines the potential of MSC for adhesion, growth, and also for maintaining a population of clonogenic cells: both a basal medium and a supplement influence these parameters. It is important to note that ready-to-use commercial media fit to MSC obtained from various sources differently. Media can cause negative effects up to early cell aging or termination of growth in the earliest passages for certain MSC type. In addition, some cell culture media can be positively selective for specific MSC subpopulations. This feature is important as the composition of MSC population might affect regenerative potential of MSC [24, 25]. The media can also influence MSC CM composition significantly.

We observed a substantial difference between several growth factor concentrations in MSC CM manufactured with two different media. Importantly, the variability of factor concentrations between two MSC CM reflected on their potency in vitro [26]. The presence or absence of a certain biologically active component in the culture medium can also affect the function of MSC. The addition of FGF2 to bone marrow MSC culture medium influences the expression of some membrane proteins, which contributes to morphology and differentiation potential changes [27]. Another challenging feature is an impact of starting material or sample processing during CM preparation. Such a routine procedure as washing cells with PBS can change the secretion profile of cells dramatically. Thus, the attention to auxiliary component and adequate selection of them are necessary [28].

Apart from materials used for MSC expansion and isolation, we might note the selection of cell culture approaches as a substantial factor affecting the variability of MSC functional properties. The use of bioreactors has been suggested as a promising alternative to conventional static culture flasks for MSC expansion. The advantage of 3D cultivation is more complete modeling of the natural microenvironment of MSC, which allows to retain the proliferation and differentiation potential of MSC for longer time. Besides, selected cell culture method can affect the secretion profile of MSC directly. Three-dimensional growth of bone marrow MSC culture influenced the expression of such factors as pigment epithelium-derived factor (PEDF), Galectin-1, brain-derived neurotrophic factor (BDNF), VEGF, nerve growth factor (NGF), insulin-like growth factor 1 (IGF-1), and miR-16, which are considered to be important regulators/modulators of the neurogenic and neural differentiation processes. Using CM from 3D cultured MSC induced the differentiation of a significantly higher number of human neural progenitors into neurons at different stages of maturation compared with human MSC secretome collected under 2D conditions [29].

5. Developing approaches to assess the potency of cell-free therapeutics

5.1. Legal aspects of potency tests development

The efficacy of a drug means a biological response caused by this drug in a certain dose. As part of a drug development, clinical research, and certified manufacturing, there is a need to develop and apply a standardized rapid method for assessing the potential efficacy of the drug. This technique is called a potency test. By definition of International Conference on Harmonization (ICH) [30], potency is the quantitative measure of biological activity based on the attribute of the product, which is linked to the relevant biological properties. The assay demonstrating the biological activity should be based on the intended biological effect which should ideally be related to the clinical response. This definition has been implemented by Food and Drug Administration (FDA) and European Medicines Agency (EMA).

At the step of research and development, the availability of an approved potency test ensures consistency among the results obtained by different scientific groups. While conducting clinical trials, postulating a presumptive potency test is necessary as one of the evaluated factors for determining the drug efficacy. At the registration stage, the presence of a clearly defined potency test is required by regulators. An established and valid potency test is required for drug manufacturing to check how scaling affects drug's therapeutic properties as well as the in-process testing for checking production lines as a factor that actually determines the lot release capability. The choice of a potency test should also be economically feasible. A potency test has to be quick and unambiguous in the context of drug efficacy determination at the earliest stages of lot release.

5.2. Development of potency tests for CM-based biopharmaceuticals

It should be emphasized that the development of an appropriate technique for potency tests of biopharmaceuticals based on cells and their secreted products is complicated (**Table 1**). In particular, the recently released "Alofisel" product faced the greatest difficulties at registration stage due to justifying the choice of potency test. "Early in the procedure a major objection was raised in relation to the potency assay. During the procedure the applicant provided additional data to support the suitability of the potency assay and the major" [31]. However, the parties managed to come to a common opinion on this issue, and the very first recommendation from the EMA was "The Applicant will undertake to review the data generated for the potency assay from clinical experience after suitable experience has been generated and to follow any recommendation that is issued following the review of the data assessment report objection is considered to be resolved."

Here, we will not dwell on the complexities of developing a potency test for cellular products, including those based on MSC; however, we note that FDA and EMA have at least a clear classification and regulatory framework for this category of therapeutics [32, 33]. At the same time, biopharmaceuticals based on MSC CM have not been classified by these agencies. Moreover, since the general rule for pharmaceutical certification is the presence of a defined, clearly characterized active substance, further progress in the development and registration of this category of therapeutics is bound to attention from regulatory agencies. According to many experts' opinions working in the field of MSC CM-based drug development, the most correct way is the approval of a new group of drugs called "cell-free therapeutics" with a less strict attitude to the issue of the multicomponent active substance [34]. The main obstacle for establishing the adequate potency tests for such biopharmaceuticals is an elusive nature of their mechanism of action (MOA) as well as the challenging choice of one active components between multiple cell-secreted factors. Nevertheless, the factors from CM composition might be isolated as single ones and classified as biological products. Therefore, it seems reasonable to apply the similar standards for characterization, safety, and dosage testing as well as potency evaluation for both the biologicals and CM, at least with any exceptions. Similar to biological drugs, potency test can be used for dose clarification from lot to lot. For complex biological medicinal products that cannot be fully characterized by physicochemical means, the established concept is to assign potency in units of biological activity based on the use of an international standard for biological activity. The units of biological activity are mostly traced back to an internationally adopted reference preparation (International Standard, IS). The quantitative composition and dosing recommendation of biological medicinal products for which an IS exists are expressed in international units (IUs) [35]. IS analogs could also be

Challenges in development and validation of PT	Possible strategies to overcome
Pleiotropic mode of action	1. One should choose the main mode of action (MOA) depending on pathological process. 2. PT must be disease-relevant and reflect preferred MOA. 3. Other MOAs specific to particular CM-based therapeutic must be taken into account. 4. Reproducible *in vitro* PT should be preferred. This model must reflect preferred MOA as accurate as possible.
Complex active substance	1. CM composition and its batch-to-batch variability should be carefully controlled. 2. Depending on preferred MOA, the most crucial components can be enriched.
"Batch-to-batch variability"	1. Complex of the most ubiquitous and crucial components should be defined at R&D phase to mitigate donor-to-donor variability. 2. Compliance to cGMP/GTP and cGLP.
Time consumption and high cost	Replacement of *in vivo* PT by *in vitro* PT or analysis of crucial components concentration (surrogate PT).
Lack of corresponding specific category in existing regulations (EMA, FDA, etc.)	Development of specific approach for regulation of multi-MOA and multicomponent CM-based therapeutics. Regulatory approach may take into account existing classes of innovative products: • CGTs/ATMPs (in aspect of usage of stem cells in manufacturing) • Biopharmaceuticals (in aspect of actual composition) • Blood plasma-derived therapeutics (in aspect of high heterogeneity and variability)

Abbreviations: PT, potency test; MOA, mode of action; CM, conditioned medium; R&D, research and development; cGMP, current good manufacturing practice; GTP, [current] good tissue practice; cGLP, current good laboratory practice; EMA, European Medicines Agency (European Union); FDA, Food and Drug Administration (USA); CGT, cellular and gene therapy; ATMP, advanced therapy medicinal product.

Table 1. Key challenges in the development of valid PT for CM-based cell-free therapeutics and possible ways to overcome them.

developed for the biopharmaceuticals derived from MSC CM. An important advantage of this approach is applicability of the direct rapid potency tests as well as the use of surrogate analytical and instrumental assays.

5.3. Challenges in the development of potency tests for CM-based products

However, MSC CM-based biopharmaceuticals represent not only a mixture of defined bioactive factors but a complex of multiple components produced by a specific type of cells. MSC CM mimics the beneficial effects of MSC cell therapy, and potency tests applied for corresponding cell and gene therapy products/advanced therapy medicinal products (CGT/ATMP) could also be relevant. For example, the measure of a defined cytokine like IL-10 in MSC secretome may serve as a potency test for a cell-based product with immunosuppressive activity and also could be used as a potency test for MSC CM-based biopharmaceutical with similar indications.

Thus, the new category of drugs to which MSC CM will belong should be based on its definitions at the junction of two existing regulating categories: biomedical drugs and CGT/ATMP.

Another complexity of creating and validating the potency test for MSC CM is the heterogeneity of the product from batch to batch. Many factors such as heterogeneity of donors, in vitro cell population during cultivation, and soluble factors that MSC can secrete under different conditions influence this phenomenon. In addition, one might develop rules for this biopharmaceutical by partial borrowing of available legal documents for preparations based on blood plasma [36] as these drugs are also highly heterogeneous, have uncertain active components, and their potency is difficult to be assessed. However, the most important hurdle in a potency test development is a variety of biological activities of factors secreted by MSC. Hence, there is a diversity of MOA, where extent and type depends on the area of application of MSC CM-based biopharmaceutical. For example, the angiogenic properties of MSC secretome are mediated by well-known pro-angiogenic factors; however, some of them may have another action. In addition, it is necessary to achieve the pleiotropic action of MSC CM, since many different mechanisms are involved in the regeneration of injuries.

It is also worth considering that in some cases, specific effects of MSC CM are contraindicated. For example, angiogenic effects necessary for the restoration of ischemic tissues may promote tumor development. Thus, the creation of a universal method for developing a potency test of MSC CM is questionable. The selection of a method for testing this substance should be disease-focused [37].

One can suggest the following mechanism for selection, testing, and validating the potency test for MSC CM (**Figure 1**). First, based on pathology nature, the most potentially effective MOA should be chosen. It is important to note that potency tests are available for the majority of MOA, and it might be possible to apply them for CM potency testing with minimal modifications.

5.4. Overcoming existing challenges in potency testing

Since there is no "gold standard" or sufficiently defined regulations in this field, developers of MSC CM-based therapeutics use a variety of approaches for determining the potency. To evaluate the immunomodulatory effect of MSC-secreted EV, an in vitro test based on a dose-dependent inhibition by vesicles of the proliferation of phytohemagglutinin-activated T lymphocytes was successfully used [38]. For the surrogate analysis of the immunomodulatory activity of MSC CM in the model of inflammatory organ failure, the effect of MSC CM on bacterial LPS-activated PBMC was tested. The degree of modulation correlated well with the level of IL-10 secreted by PBMC in this experimental model [39]. The subsidiary company of SteMedica, StemProtein, has successfully used two potency tests for its unique product, human fibroblast secretome dried by proprietary technology "Preservation by Vaporization." Because tissue regeneration critically depends on adequate blood supply, they used in vitro angiogenesis assays to evaluate the therapeutic potency of stem cell factors. They routinely monitored the concentrations of VEGF, HGF, interleukin 6 (IL-6), chemokine C-C motif ligand 2 (CCL2), C-X-C motif chemokine 5 (CXCL5),

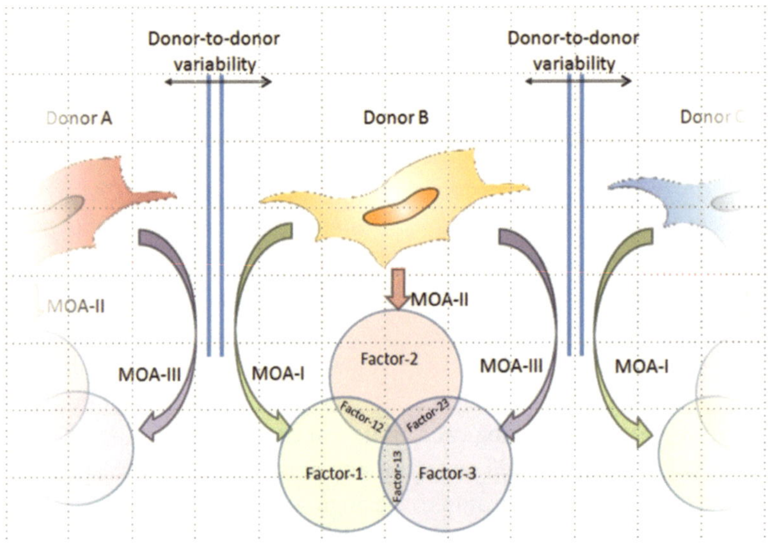

Figure 1. Schematic reflecting multicomponent multi-MOA nature of MSC and effects of factors secreted by them. A detailed description is provided in the subsequent text. Abbreviations: MOA, mode of action; MSC, mesenchymal stromal cells.

and interleukin 8 (CXCL8) in the product, as published literature has identified the important biological activity of these growth factors, cytokines, and chemokines [40, 41]. MultiStem also successfully used an analogous in vitro angiogenic test of biological activity, and also showed that three factors—VEGF, CXCL8, and CXCL5—are the crucial factors for the angiogenic activity of the secretome. The depletion of any of them drops the angiogenic effect of the secretome. Concentrations of each of the factors can be used as a threshold for the lot release [42]. Based on the literature data and guidelines as well as on our own experimental results, we provided rationalization for nomenclature and methods of quality control for human adipose-derived MSC CM developed for tissue reparation and regeneration on "Specific activity." As the most important type of cells involved in tissue repair and regeneration after injury are fibroblasts, one of the models for MSC CM potency measurement was the assessment of human skin fibroblasts migration in the model of the scratch assay. In this regard that angiogenesis is also an indispensable process for the successful regeneration of tissues, we additionally used a model of human endothelial cells direct migration upon MSC CM gradient [26].

Despite direct in vitro or in vivo biological activity tests seem to be more informative, they demonstrate several substantial disadvantages. The main challenge is to render some injury-specific conditions in model objects. Many in vivo studies in the fields of oncology and adaptive immunity conducted on rodents have faced this problem. In accordance with the provisions of the European Convention for the Protection of Vertebrate Animals Used for Experimental and Other Scientific Purposes and Directive 2010/63/EU on protection of animals used for scientific purposes, the 3R principles (replacement, reduction, and refinement) should be applied to production and control testing of medicinal products. [43]. Last but not the least, it is rational to take into account a high cost of these types of potency test.

As CM action is mediated by the soluble factors, the development of a surrogate test based on the correlations between defined factor concentration (e.g., measured by immunoassay) and potency seems to be reasonable. It is necessary to analyze secretome profiles of cells from a large number of donors in order to detect the most robust and relevant active factors in CM concerning current MOA. The molecules selected for this analysis should be the most significant for maintenance of the selected MOA, and less significant for another MOA. In **Figure 1**, if someone selects MOA-II as pivotal one, he should firstly consider factor-2 as the candidate for the surrogate test. Factor-12 and factor-23, which apart from MOA-II are involved in MOA-I and MOA-III, respectively, should be chosen only if their levels are crucial for the MOA-II potential.

6. Conclusion

This chapter is dedicated to a novel class of biopharmaceuticals based on secretory components of MSC as products for regenerative medicine. CM-based cell-free therapeutics comprise multicomponent mixture with multiple targets and pleiotropic effects. These biopharmaceuticals reproduce many benefits of the rapidly developing cell therapy products. However, the use of cells might be complicated due to ectopic transplantation, tumorigenesis, and immune system reactions. MSC secretome is devoid of cell therapy side effects and has substantial advantages in manufacture, storage, and standardization making it a promising type of biopharmaceuticals.

We paid attention to safe and effective MSC CM-based cell-free therapeutics manufacturing conception. We have discussed several challenges concerning donor-associated variability, cell isolation procedure, optimal protocols for manufacturing and quality control, and lack of key regulatory decisions that must be overcome prior to the wide-scale clinical translation of such therapeutics. To reach the best safety and efficacy marks, developers could apply a system-wide approach to disease model analysis considering the principal mechanisms of tissue reparation and regeneration processes. In addition, it is rational to develop appropriate donor selection criteria that can help to involve only a suitable starting material to manufacturing process. Preventing the lot-to-lot variability together with improved efficacy could be facilitated by a relevant potency test development and validation required for the drug-quality control. The use of rational approach to the choice of MOA might help to relieve development and conduction of a potency test by transition to more simple surrogate approach. In addition, implementing of these approaches into practice would help to develop novel legal potency test guidelines for cell-free therapeutics with unambiguous rules and examples.

Funding information

The reported study was funded by RFBR according to the research project No. 18-315-00403 and carried out within the state assignment of Lomonosov MSU.

Author details

Georgy D. Sagaradze[1,2], Peter P. Nimiritsky[1,2], Zhanna A. Akopyan[1,2], Pavel I. Makarevich[1,2]* and Anastasia Yu. Efimenko[1,2]

*Address all correspondence to: pmakarevich@mc.msu.ru

1 Institute for Regenerative Medicine, Medical Research and Education Center, Lomonosov, Moscow State University, Moscow, Russian Federation

2 Faculty of Medicine, Lomonosov Moscow State University, Moscow, Russian Federation

References

[1] Crane GM, Jeffery E, Morrison SJ. Adult haematopoietic stem cell niches. Nature Reviews. Immunology. 2017;**17**(9):573-590. DOI: 10.1038/nri.2017.53

[2] Méndez-Ferrer S, Michurina TV, Ferraro F, Mazloom AR, MacArthur BD, Lira SA, et al. Mesenchymal and haematopoietic stem cells form a unique bone marrow niche. Nature. 2010;**466**(7308):829-834. DOI: 10.1038/nature09262

[3] Sacchetti B, Funari A, Michienzi S, Di Cesare S, Piersanti S, Saggio I, et al. Self-renewing osteoprogenitors in bone marrow sinusoids can organize a hematopoietic microenvironment. Cell. 2007;**131**(2):324-336. DOI: 10.1016/J.CELL.2007.08.025

[4] Gotts JE, Matthay MA. Mesenchymal stem cells and the stem cell niche: A new chapter. American Journal of Physiology. Lung Cellular and Molecular Physiology. 2012; **302**(11):L1147-L1149. DOI: 10.1152/ajplung.00122.2012

[5] Vizoso F, Eiro N, Cid S, Schneider J, Perez-Fernandez R. Mesenchymal stem cell secretome: Toward cell-free therapeutic strategies in regenerative medicine. International Journal of Molecular Sciences. 2017;**18**(12):1852. DOI: 10.3390/ijms18091852

[6] Kalinina N, Kharlampieva D, Loguinova M, Butenko I, Pobeguts O, Efimenko A, et al. Characterization of secretomes provides evidence for adipose-derived mesenchymal stromal cells subtypes. Stem Cell Research & Therapy. 2015;**6**(1):221. DOI: 10.1186/s13287-015-0209-8

[7] Baglio SR, Rooijers K, Koppers-Lalic D, Verweij FJ, Pérez Lanzón M, Zini N, et al. Human bone marrow- and adipose-mesenchymal stem cells secrete exosomes enriched in distinctive miRNA and tRNA species. Stem Cell Research & Therapy. 2015;**6**(1):127. DOI: 10.1186/s13287-015-0116-z

[8] Valtieri M, Sorrentino A. The mesenchymal stromal cell contribution to homeostasis. Journal of Cellular Physiology. 2008;**217**(2):296-300. DOI: 10.1002/jcp.21521

[9] Montagnani S, Rueger MA, Hosoda T, Nurzynska D. Adult stem cells in tissue maintenance and regeneration. Stem Cells International. 2016;**2016**:1-2. DOI: 10.1155/2016/7362879

[10] Lai RC, Arslan F, Lee MM, Sze NSK, Choo A, Chen TS, et al. Exosome secreted by MSC reduces myocardial ischemia/reperfusion injury. Stem Cell Research. 2010;**4**(3):214-222. DOI: 10.1016/J.SCR.2009.12.003

[11] Bhang SH, Lee S, Shin JY, Lee TJ, Jang HK, Kim BS. Efficacious and clinically relevant conditioned medium of human adipose-derived stem cells for therapeutic angiogenesis. Molecular Therapy. 2014;**22**(4):862-872. DOI: 10.1038/mt.2013.301

[12] Liu S, Zhou J, Zhang X, Liu Y, Chen J, Hu B, et al. Strategies to optimize adult stem cell therapy for tissue regeneration. International Journal of Molecular Sciences. 2016; **17**(6):982. DOI: 10.3390/ijms17060982

[13] Nguyen PK, Neofytou E, Rhee J-W, Wu JC. Potential strategies to address the major clinical barriers facing stem cell regenerative therapy for cardiovascular disease. JAMA Cardiology. 2016;**1**(8):953. DOI: 10.1001/jamacardio.2016.2750

[14] Herberts CA, Kwa MS, Hermsen HP. Risk factors in the development of stem cell therapy. Journal of Translational Medicine. 2011;**9**(1):29. DOI: 10.1186/1479-5876-9-29

[15] Schimke MM, Marozin S, Lepperdinger G. Patient-specific age: The other side of the coin in advanced mesenchymal stem cell therapy. Frontiers in Physiology. 2015;**6**:362. DOI: 10.3389/fphys.2015.00362

[16] Efimenko A, Dzhoyashvili N, Kalinina N, Kochegura T, Akchurin R, Tkachuk V, et al. Adipose-derived mesenchymal stromal cells from aged patients with coronary artery disease keep mesenchymal stromal cell properties but exhibit characteristics of aging and have impaired angiogenic potential. Stem Cells Translational Medicine. 2014;**3**(1):32-41. DOI: 10.5966/sctm.2013-0014

[17] Efimenko A, Starostina E, Kalinina N, Stolzing A. Angiogenic properties of aged adipose derived mesenchymal stem cells after hypoxic conditioning. Journal of Translational Medicine. 2011;**9**(1):10. DOI: 10.1186/1479-5876-9-10

[18] Kizilay Mancini O, Shum-Tim D, Stochaj U, Correa JA, Colmegna I. Age, atherosclerosis and type 2 diabetes reduce human mesenchymal stromal cell-mediated T-cell suppression. Stem Cell Research & Therapy. 2015;**6**(1):140. DOI: 10.1186/s13287-015-0127-9

[19] Mohd Ali N, Boo L, Yeap SK, Ky H, Satharasinghe DA, Liew WC, et al. Probable impact of age and hypoxia on proliferation and microRNA expression profile of bone marrow-derived human mesenchymal stem cells. PeerJ [Internet]. 2016;**14**(4):e1536. DOI: 10.7717/peerj.1536

[20] Peffers MJ, Collins J, Fang Y, Goljanek-Whysall K, Rushton M, Loughlin J, Proctor C, Clegg PD. Age-related changes in mesenchymal stem cells identified using a multi-omics approach. European Cells & Materials. 2016;**31**:136-159. DOI: 10.22203/eCM.v031a10

[21] Siegel G, Kluba T, Hermanutz-Klein U, Bieback K, Northoff H, Schäfer R. Phenotype, donor age and gender affect function of human bone marrow-derived mesenchymal stromal cells. BMC Medicine. 2013;**11**(1):146. DOI: 10.1186/1741-7015-11-146

[22] Pasanen I, Pietilä M, Lehtonen S, Lehtilahti E, Hakkarainen T, Blanco Sequeiros R, et al. Mesenchymal stromal cells from female donors enhance breast cancer cell proliferation in vitro. Oncology. 2015;**88**(4):214-225. DOI: 10.1159/000368556

[23] Strioga M, Viswanathan S, Darinskas A, Slaby O, Michalek J. Same or not the same? Comparison of adipose tissue-derived versus bone marrow-derived mesenchymal stem and stromal cells. Stem Cells and Development. 2012;**21**(14):2724-2752. DOI: 10.1089/scd.2011.0722

[24] Al-Saqi SH, Saliem M, Asikainen S, et al. Defined serum-free media for in vitro expansion of adipose-derived mesenchymal stem cells. Cytotherapy. 2014;**16**(7):915-926. DOI: 10.1016/j.jcyt.2014.02.006

[25] Riis S, Nielsen FM, Pennisi CP, Zachar V, Fink T. Comparative analysis of media and supplements on initiation and expansion of adipose-derived stem cells. Stem Cells Translational Medicine. 2016;**5**(3):314-324. DOI: 10.5966/sctm.2015-0148

[26] Sagaradze GD, Grigorieva OA, Efimenko AY, Chaplenko AA, Suslina SN, Sysoeva VY, et al. Therapeutic potential of human mesenchymal stromal cells secreted components: A problem with standartization. Biomeditsinskaya Khimiya. 2015;**61**(6):750-759. DOI: 10.18097/PBMC20156106750

[27] Lee SK, Kim Y, Kim S-S, Lee JH, Cho K, Lee SS, et al. Differential expression of cell surface proteins in human bone marrow mesenchymal stem cells cultured with or without basic fibroblast growth factor containing medium. Proteomics. 2009;**9**(18):4389-4405. DOI: 10.1002/pmic.200900165

[28] Clabaut A, Grare C, Léger T, Hardouin P, Broux O. Variations of secretome profiles according to conditioned medium preparation: The example of human mesenchymal stem cell-derived adipocytes. Electrophoresis. 2015;**36**(20):2587-2593. DOI: 10.1002/elps.201500086

[29] Teixeira FG, Panchalingam KM, Assunção-Silva R, Serra SC, Mendes-Pinheiro B, Patrício P, et al. Modulation of the mesenchymal stem cell secretome using computer-controlled bioreactors: Impact on neuronal cell proliferation, survival and differentiation. Scientific Reports. 2016;**6**(1):27791. DOI: 10.1038/srep27791

[30] Teasdale A, Elder DP, Nims RW, editors. ICH Quality Guidelines: An Implementation Guide. Chichester: Wiley; 2017. 736 p. ISBN: 978-1-118-97111-6

[31] European Medicines Agency, Committee for Medicinal Products for Human Use (CHMP). Assessment Report Alofisel [Internet]. 2017. Available from: http://www.ema.europa.eu/docs/en_GB/document_library/EPAR_-_Public_assessment_report/human/004258/WC500246476.pdf [Accessed: 2018-04-15]

[32] U.S. Department of Health and Human Services, Food and Drug Administration, Center for Biologics Evaluation and Research. Guidance for industry potency tests for cellular and gene. Federal Register [Internet]. 2011. Available from: https://www.fda.gov/downloads/BiologicsBloodVaccines/GuidanceComplianceRegulatoryInformation/Guidances/CellularandGeneTherapy/UCM243392.pdf [Accessed: 2018-05-07]

[33] The European Parliament and The Council of The European Union. Regulation (EC) No. 1394/2007 of 13 November 2007 on advanced therapy medicinal products and amending

directive 2001/83/EC and Regulation (EC) No. 726/2004. Official Journal of the European Union [Internet]. 2007. Available from: https://ec.europa.eu/health/sites/health/files/files/eudralex/vol-1/reg_2007_1394/reg_2007_1394_en.pdf [Accessed: 2018-05-07]

[34] Bersenev A. Commercialization of stem cell secretome [Internet]. 2015. Available from: http://stemcellassays.com/2015/04/commercialization-stem-cell-secretome/ [Accessed: 2018-05-07]

[35] European Medicines Agency, Committee for Medicinal Products for Human Use (CHMP). Guideline on the declaration of the quantitative composition/potency labelling of biological medicinal products that contain modified proteins as active substance. EMA Guideline [Internet]. 2014. Available from: http://www.ema.europa.eu/docs/en_GB/document_library/Scientific_guideline/2014/03/WC500163595.pdf [Accessed: 2018-04-15]

[36] European Medicines Agency, Committee for Medicinal Products for Human Use (CHMP). Guideline on plasma-derived medicinal products. EMA Guideline [Internet]. 2011. Available from: http://www.ema.europa.eu/docs/en_GB/document_library/Scientific_guideline/2011/07/WC500109627.pdf [Accessed: 2018-05-07]

[37] Gimona M, Pachler K, Laner-Plamberger S, Schallmoser K, Rohde E. Manufacturing of human extracellular vesicle-based therapeutics for clinical use. International Journal of Molecular Sciences. 2017;**18**(6):1190. DOI: 10.3390/ijms18061190

[38] Pachler K, Ketterl N, Desgeorges A, Dunai Z, Laner-Plamberger S, Streif D, et al. An in vitro potency assay for monitoring the immunomodulatory potential of stromal cell-derived extracellular vesicles. International Journal of Molecular Sciences. 2017;**18**(7):1413. DOI: 10.3390/ijms18071413

[39] Jiao J, Milwid JM, Yarmush ML, Parekkadan BA. Mesenchymal stem cell potency assay. In: Cuturi MC, Anegon I, editors. Suppression and Regulation of Immune Responses. Totowa, NJ: Humana Press; 2010. pp. 221-231. DOI: 10.1007/978-1-60761-869-0_16

[40] StemProtein. Stem cell factors web-page [Internet]. Available from: http://stemprotein.com/ [Accessed: 2018-04-15]

[41] Newman AC, Nakatsu MN, Chou W, Gershon PD, Hughes CCW. The requirement for fibroblasts in angiogenesis: Fibroblast-derived matrix proteins are essential for endothelial cell lumen formation. Molecular Biology of the Cell. 2011;**22**(20):3791-3800. DOI: 10.1091/mbc.E11-05-0393

[42] Lehman N, Cutrone R, Raber A, Perry R, Van't Hof W, Deans R, et al. Development of a surrogate angiogenic potency assay for clinical-grade stem cell production. Cytotherapy. 2012;**14**(8):994-1004. DOI: 10.3109/14653249.2012.688945

[43] European Medicines Agency. Statement of the EMA position on the application of the 3Rs (replacement, reduction and refinement) in the regulatory testing of human and veterinary medicinal products [Internet]. 2011. Available from: http://www.ema.europa.eu/docs/en_GB/document_library/Other/2011/10/WC500115625.pdf [Accessed: 2018-04-15]

Section 4

Application

Chapter 4

Impact of Immunotherapy in the Treatment of Glioblastoma

Jessica Silva, Ana Miranda, João Sousa,
Alberto Pais and Carla Vitorino

Additional information is available at the end of the chapter

http://dx.doi.org/10.5772/intechopen.78603

Abstract

Glioblastoma multiforme (GBM) is the most common and aggressive primary malignant brain tumor. Despite the efforts developed in the respective treatment, consisting of maximal surgical resection followed by adjuvant radiotherapy and chemotherapy, the prognosis remains very poor. This may be partly related to the resistance of GBM cells and their infiltrative and invasive nature into the surrounding brain tissue. Therefore, newer and challenging alternative approaches for the treatment have emerged, including immunotherapy. This anticancer therapy, based on the stimulation of the host's immune system, has been currently investigated and several advances in the clinical trial stage have already been reached. Immunotherapeutic strategies comprise a set of modalities, including vaccines (cell-free and cell-based), chimeric antigen receptor (CAR) T-cell therapy, immune checkpoint inhibitors, monoclonal antibodies (mAbs), and oncolytic viruses (OVs). In this chapter, we will review the principal concepts and the recent progress in immunotherapy for GBM.

Keywords: glioblastoma multiforme, immunotherapy, vaccine, antigen, dendritic cell, clinical trial

1. Introduction

Glioblastoma multiforme (GBM), histologically a World Health Organization (WHO) grade IV glioma, is the most common and aggressive malignant brain tumor, accounting for approximately 45–50% of all primary malignant brain tumors. Despite the efforts developed by its current standard therapy (maximal surgical tumor resection followed by concomitant radiotherapy plus temozolomide (TMZ) chemotherapy), GBM remains an incurable disease with a poor prognosis that attains a median survival of 14.6 months and a mean survival rate of 0.05–4.7% at 5 years, which is partially due to its heterogeneous and invasive nature as well as to the tumor resistance [1–3]. In addition, it is well-known that the protective nature of the blood–brain barrier (BBB) limits the entry of therapeutic agents into the brain and consequently hampers the success of therapies [4].

Recently, new and promising immunotherapeutic approaches have emerged and evidenced a great impact in GBM treatment, harnessing the ability of the host's immune system to induce or enhance antitumor responses [2, 5]. These immunotherapeutic strategies are related with both active immunotherapy, such as vaccines (cell-free and cell-based), and passive immunotherapy, namely monoclonal antibodies (mAbs), immune checkpoint inhibitors, chimeric antigen receptor (CAR) T-cell therapy and oncolytic viruses (OVs). Despite the presence of the BBB, such strategies can be successful by considering some key points. If immunotherapy is intended to be given intravenously, the BBB is effectively a problem, but likely to be exceeded. On the one hand, it is noteworthy that patients with GBM tend to have a fenestrated endothelium with BBB disruption, which will possibly facilitate the passage of immunotherapeutic cells. On the other hand, there are already mechanisms to induce a reversible BBB opening with a transiently increase in the respective permeability. Nonetheless, there is currently an easier and more effective approach, which consists of direct intracranial injection of immunotherapeutic agents, thus overcoming the problems associated with the BBB [4, 6].

Regardless the low number of clinical trials (CT) that are completed to date, the early results reached for all of these strategies are generally related with positive patient outcomes, which has increased the interest in proceeding with the investigations. This chapter provides a brief description and the currently ongoing CT of all of these therapies, with particular emphasis on vaccines. In fact, vaccination represents a valuable therapeutic option in cancer since it can induce widespread and sustained antitumor effects, with less toxicity than standard chemotherapy [7, 8].

2. The spectrum of vaccine strategies in glioblastoma

Contrary to chemotherapy and passive immunotherapy, vaccination does not have a direct antitumor effect, but rather boosts the immune system to destroy tumor cells [9]. More precisely, vaccines aim at inducing tumor-specific immune responses, mainly based on $CD8^+$ cytotoxic T lymphocytes (CTL), which are specific to tumor antigens [10]. According to the strategy used to present the antigens to the immune system, cancer vaccines can be divided mainly in two groups, cell-free or cell-based vaccines [11].

2.1. Cell-free vaccines

Treatment with cell-free vaccines consists on direct inoculation of single or multi antigens, later presented to host antigen-presenting cell (APC) that, upon such stimulation, migrate to lymph nodes where they boost immune response. In this group are included a peptide, multipeptide, and heat-shock protein (HSP) vaccines, whose applicability has already been developed for GBM [11–13].

2.1.1. *Peptide and multipeptide vaccines*

Cancer peptide vaccines take advantage of peptides to trigger a pharmacological activity through the mobilization of the immune system against tumor antigens [13]. Investigating the expression profile of antigens in human GBM thus becomes the most important step in the process of developing vaccine-directed immunotherapy [14]. In fact, multiple glioma-related antigens have been identified and even tested in vaccine trials over the last years, but only a few reached promising results given the known variable expression patterns of proteins/antigen among GBM patients [14, 15]. These vaccines may incorporate a single or multiple, long or short peptides acting as tumor antigens, which are often coupled to carrier proteins in order to potentiate their immunogenicity [15, 16]. Although being a recent treatment modality in oncology, GBM has already a varied range of successfully proven vaccines, many of them peptide/multipeptide vaccines [11].

Considering the frequent amplification of epidermal growth factor receptor (EGFR) and its active mutant EGFRvIII in GBM, many researchers have focused their works on developing EGFRvIII vaccines with remarkable clinical results. For instance, rindopepimut (also called Rintega® and CDX-110) was subjected to a number of phase I/II CT since its introduction (VICTORI, pediatric pontine glioma pilot study (NCT01130077), ACTIVATE (NCT00643097), ACT II, ACT III (NCT00458601), and ReACT (NCT01498328)), where its clinical efficacy was clearly shown in patients with GBM. Such vaccination resulted in prolonged progression-free and overall survival (OS) with no safety concerns. However, a phase III CT (ACT IV (NCT01480479)) with rindopepimut was discontinued since the study failed to meet its primary OS endpoint [7, 17, 18]. Another example is a live attenuated *Listeria*-based vaccine (ADU-623) expressing both EGFRvIII and NY-ESO-1 antigens, which is currently being tested in patients with recurrent GBM through a phase I CT (NCT01967758) [11, 18].

Despite the increased interest in EGFRvIII, other antigens have been considered for the investigation of immunotherapy in GBM, with emphasis on SurVaxM, PEPIDH1M, and DSP-7888 vaccines. SVN53-67/M57 (SurVaxM), a peptide vaccine derived from survivin, not only has revealed promising results in preclinical studies with GL261-bearing mice but has also been investigated in CT (phase II so far (NCT02455557)) [11, 18, 19]. Since isocitrate dehydrogenase 1 (IDH1) is an enzyme commonly mutated in GBM, it has been developed IDH1 peptide vaccines for patients with glioma positive for IDH1 R132H mutation (presented in 5–12% of GBMs). Currently, two phase I CT are being conducted for that purpose, called RESIST trial (NCT02193347) with PEPIDH1M vaccine and NOA-16 (NCT02454634), both of which target patients with IDH1R132H-mutated gliomas [15, 20]. Another developing peptide vaccine uses the tumor-associated antigens (TAA) Wilm's tumor protein-1 (WT-1), recognized as an oncogene expressed in GBM responsible for tumor growth. WT1 peptide vaccination has been investigated through several phases I/II CT, alone or in combination with other therapeutics, including TMZ. Overall, the results of these WT1-based vaccines have been positive, confirming their safety profile along with good clinical responses. By way of example, DSP-7888 vaccine revealed to induce a specific CTL and helper T-lymphocyte-mediated immune responses against WT1 expressing GBM, in a phase I CT (NCT02498665) [11, 18].

When not one but several antigens are incorporated in the same vaccine, multi-peptide vaccines are obtained as the case of IMA950, SL-701, and ERC-1671 vaccines. In fact, combining multiple peptides in a single mixture may offer therapeutic advantages bearing in mind the heterogeneous gene expression profiles in different GBM [15, 21]. IMA950 is a vaccine encompassing 11 peptides naturally presented in GBM tissue (brevican; chondroitin sulfate proteoglycan 4; fatty acid binding protein 7, brain; insulin-like growth factor 2 mRNA binding protein 3; neuroligin 4, X-linked; neuronal cell adhesion molecule; protein tyrosine phosphatase, receptor-type, Z polypeptide 1; tenascin C; Met proto-oncogene; baculoviral inhibitor of apoptosis protein repeat-containing 5; and hepatitis B virus core antigen). This multipeptide vaccine has been subjected to numerous phase I/II CT (NCT02924038, NCT01920191, NCT01403285, and NCT01222221), alone or combined with other therapies, whose results are still somewhat inconclusive as to its clinical efficacy [11, 18]. Another case, the SL-701 vaccine composed of 3 peptides (a highly immunogenic mutant to target survivin, interleukin-13 receptor α-2 (IL-13Rα2), and ephrin A2) was investigated in adults with recurrent GBM through a phase I/II CT (NCT02078648), although the results have not yet been disclosed [11, 14, 18]. A slightly more complex vaccine concerns ERC-1671 (Gliovac) since it uses a combination of allogeneic tumor cells (derived from three different GBM donors), autologous GBM tumor cells (resultant from resected tumor of the patient) and GBM tumor lysates. Given the notable results obtained from the first clinical studies, this multi-peptide vaccine moved toward a phase II CT (NCT01903330), being examined in recurrent, bevacizumab naive GBM patients [11]. As it is well-known, O^6-methylguanin-DNA-methyltransferase (MGMT) unmethylated GBM is correlated with TMZ resistance and worse prognosis of the tumor [22]. Such evidence led to the development of a personalized neoantigen cancer vaccine (NeoVax), which is currently being examined in a phase I CT (NCT03422094) along with radiotherapy in newly diagnosed GBM with exclusively unmethylated MGMT promoters [18].

2.1.2. Heat-shock protein (HSP) vaccines

HSPs act as chaperones for intracellular proteins, so they have the ability to bind, fold and chaperone an antigenic representation of the cells from which they are originated. Based on this fact, HSPs isolated and purified from a patient's resected tumor can be subsequently reinfused, and then they will promote the presentation of antigenic peptides to APCs, which elicit antigen-specific CTL responses [11, 18]. Among the proteins of the HSP family, expressed in GBM, HSP70 and HSP90 stand out. Despite the dysregulation of these HSP families being reported to play a critical role in tumor proliferation, invasiveness, and metastasis, in addition to suppression of apoptosis, HSP70 and HSP90 have also shown ability to bind antigenic peptides, which can elicit tumor rejection responses [23]. HSP70 family inhibits cell stress-induced apoptotic pathways, facilitates protein folding, and guides protein transport across membranes, while HSP90 mainly assists in protein folding, protein stabilization, and peptide loading onto major histocompatibility complex (MHC) class I molecules. Particularly, HSP90 was found to bind to EGFRvIII, FAK, AKT, hTERT, p53, cdk4, MAPK, and PI3K in GBM, which are involved in key tumor initiation and proliferation signaling pathways. Although the studies have been conducted for other types of tumors, it is believed that the same may occur with GBM, with HSP presenting tumor-specific antigens to stimulate antitumor immune responses [11, 24, 25]. Autologous tumor-derived HSP-peptide complex 96 (HSPPC-96) have generated great interest over the last few years, reason why it has been the most used in HSP vaccine trials. In fact, HSPPC-96 has been extensively explored in several phases I/II CT (NCT02722512, NCT00905060, NCT01814813, NCT00293423, and among others), most of them for GBM patients, inducing strong tumor-specific immune responses with the improved median OS [11, 14, 18, 26].

2.2. Cell-based vaccines

Contrary to the vaccines previously presented, cell-based vaccines (as the name itself indicates) first resort to APCs *ex vivo*, most often dendritic cells (DCs) extracted from the patient, loading them with tumor antigens. After activation, they are injected into the host, presenting the antigens to naive T cells of the adaptive immune system [11, 27].

2.2.1. Dendritic cells (DCs) vaccines

As is already known, DC are considered the optimal APC of the immune system, due to their ability to stimulate T and B lymphocytes, in addition to promoting natural killer (NK) T cells activation [28, 29]. As such, a wide range of antigen sources has been explored for pulsing of DC, and include tumor peptides, autologous tumor lysates, tumor-derived mRNA (messenger RNA), glioblastoma stem cells (GSCs) and viral antigens. All of these strategies have already been properly tested in GBM, proving to be immunogenic with very promising outcomes [5, 11, 14, 15, 28].

Referring to tumor peptide-loaded DCs, we here present the two most important so far: autologous DC pulsed with an EGFRvIII peptide conjugated with keyhole limpet hemocyanin (PEPvIII-KLH), and the ICT-107 autologous vaccine [11]. The latter concerns patient DCs pulsed with six synthetic TAAs (AIM-2, MAGE1, TRP-2, gp100, HER2/neu, and IL-13Rα2, four of which are considered GSC-associated, and whose results obtained in phase I/II CT (NCT01280552) are quite encouraging for the ongoing phase III CT (NCT02546102) in GBM [5, 11, 14]. As a matter of fact, ICT-107 is also considered a tumor stem cell vaccine. It should be recalled that GBM possesses a small subpopulation of self-renewing, tumorigenic GSC, which drive invasive tumor growth and therapeutic resistance. Among the biomarkers studied, CD133 has been used extensively to identify and isolate tumor stem cells, given its overexpression on these malignant cells [7, 18, 30]. In this sense, ICT-107 vaccine was found to decrease CD133$^+$ cells from recurrent GBM; moreover, the tumor stem cell vaccine ICT-121 consists of autologous DC pulsed with purified peptides from CD133, whose safety and clinical response will be assessed in a phase I CT now ongoing (NCT02049489) [18]. Still on the stemness, another way to take advantage of GSC is to develop tumor-derived mRNA-loaded DCs vaccines. In this case, autologous GSC cultures are established from resected tumor, followed by isolation of RNA and amplification of mRNA, then transfected into DC [31, 32]. As such, a phase I CT (NCT00890032) studied CD133+ autologous brain tumor stem cell (BTSC) mRNA-loaded DC in patients with recurrent GBM, which revealed to be safe, feasible and well-tolerated [32].

An alternative approach involves using tumor cell lysates-loaded DCs, such as DCVax®-L vaccine in which cellular fragments (derived from the patient's own resected tumor) are pulsed into DCs. In fact, this technique offers the advantage of collecting a broad spectrum of patients' tumor antigens, known and unknown (given the heterogeneity of antigen expression among gliomas), thus triggering a polyclonal immune response [11, 14, 28, 33]. DCVax®-L, one of the most promising vaccines for GBM, consists of an autologous DC vaccine that is currently under evaluation in a phase III CT (NCT00045968). Previous studies (phase I/II CT) have proved its safety profile, also demonstrating that vaccine can increase progression-free and OS in newly diagnosed GBM (2 out of 39 patients survived more than 10 years) [2, 18, 34].

It has been reported that most GBM express exclusive human cytomegalovirus (CMV) proteins, as for example IE1, US28, pp65, gB, HCMV IL-10, and pp28. Such evidence made possible the use of immunodominant CMV antigens to produce viral antigen-loaded DCs, aimed at treating GBM patients [14, 15]. Exciting results were obtained in a study with patient-derived DCs pulsed with CMV pp65 RNA since the stimulation of CMV pp65-specific cytotoxic T cells resulted in recognition and destruction of autologous GBM tumor cells in an antigen-specific manner [35]. In the wake of this outcome, a phase II CT (NCT02366728) is currently ongoing testing the CMV pp65 RNA-pulsed autologous DC vaccine along with tetanus/diphtheria toxoid helper vaccine, for newly diagnosed GBM patients [18]. In addition, the DC vaccine PEP-CMV comprises two peptides, derived from human pp65 and gB, and has been investigated in some phase I CTs (NCT01854099, NCT02864368, and NCT03299309) without published results so far [7, 15].

2.2.2. Human umbilical vein endothelial cell (HUVEC) vaccines

Less commonly used in vaccines, but also with ongoing trials for GBM, are the glutaraldehyde-fixed human umbilical vein endothelial cells (HUVECs). [14, 36]. As it is well known, angiogenesis is a hallmark of GBM that facilitates tumor progression and invasiveness. Based on that, HUVEC vaccination consists of an endovascular targeting immunotherapy intended to trigger an antiangiogenic response, upon presentation of HUVEC antigen to the immune system [14, 37]. To the best of our knowledge, only two preliminary CT was conducted with HUVEC vaccines for recurrent GBM patients, whose clinical outcomes were promising without serious adverse events associated [14, 36, 38]. In addition, an interesting *in vivo* study assessed the effect of a combined vaccine, prepared from GBM and endothelial cells, on glioma-bearing mice. While tumor growth inhibition was seen only in the preventive use of the combined vaccine, a significantly decrease in vessel account was verified in the tumor upon the therapeutic experiment with that vaccine [37].

2.2.3. Autologous formalin-fixed tumor vaccines (AFTVs)

Last but not least, are whole tumor cell vaccines, which use autologous formalin-fixed tumor fragments obtained from surgical removal to trigger *in vivo* antigen-specific CTL responses [39, 40].

Actually, formalin fixation technique has been used since it allows admirable preservation of tissue morphology, and consequently, the antigenicity of tumor cells [14, 40]. A CT with an autologous formalin-fixed tumor vaccine (AFTV) being tested in 12 primary GBM patients demonstrated the safety and viability of the vaccine, along with promising clinical responses that were also achieved [40]. Another study, phase I/IIa CT, examined the impact of an AFTV concomitant with radiotherapy in 22 resected patients with newly diagnosed GBM. Such trial resulted in median OS of 19.8 months with an actuarial 2-year survival rate of 40%, in addition to not reporting serious adverse events [39]. Interestingly, an immunotherapy strategy combining cellular vaccines (prepared from autologous GL261 murine glioma cells and F-2 murine endothelial cells) was tested on glioma-bearing mice. Such preclinical study revealed that combined vaccine significantly decreased tumor growth and vessel account, thus representing an expecting strategy capable to target both GBM cells and their microenvironment [37].

2.3. Advantages and disadvantages of cell-free and cell-based vaccines

Throughout this chapter, several candidate vaccine approaches are presented for GBM treatment. Although most of them have demonstrated safety and clinical benefit in different

Strategy	Advantages	Disadvantages
Cell-free vaccines	• Easy to synthethize, purify, produce and standardize; [16, 41, 42] • Cost-effective approach; [41] • Safe with no biological contamination (in case of synthetic peptides); [42] • Stable in storage; [16] • Possibility of selecting one or more antigens (stimulation of an specific immune response); [16, 41] • Fully-defined composition; • Low risk of allergic and auto imune responses, as well as of oncogenicity effects [41, 42]	• Prior and proper identification of immunogenic epitope(s); [41] • Existence of antigen-loss tumor variants; [16] • MHC restriction; [41] • Lack of helper activity and weak presentation of antigen by endogenous APC (contrary to the cross-presentation by DC); [16] • Instability of peptides *in vivo* being rapidly degraded by peptidases [16]
Cell-based vaccines	• Bypass the endogenous DC dysfunction in cancer patients; [43] • Cross-presentation of exogenous antigens by DC; [44] • Great ability of DC to prime T cells to attack the tumor; [44] • AFTV provide the entire spectrum of TAAs with no need to select the most proper antigen to target the tumor; [45] • Safe, multivalent and patient-specific [12]	• High production costs; [42] • Quality concerns due to the manufacture highly variable; [12, 42] • Poor immunogenicity of the tumor cell themselves; [12] • Most of them are restricted to patients with a resectable tumor; [42, 46] • Some failure rate associated with culture of autologous tumor cells [46]

MHC: major histocompatibility complex; APC: antigen-presenting cell; DC: dendritic cell; TAA: tumor-associated antigens; AFTV: autologous formalin-fixed tumor vaccine.

Table 1. Overall assessment of cell-free and cell-based vaccines.

preclinical and clinical studies, it is essential to understand some intrinsic advantages and disadvantages of cell-free and cell-based vaccines in cancer therapy (**Table 1**).

3. Other immunotherapeutic strategies

Equally important, immunotherapeutic approaches, such as monoclonal antibodies, immune checkpoint inhibitors, adoptive T-cell therapy, CAR T-cell therapy and oncolytic viruses, have been investigated in the treatment of GBM [47]. Some related clinical data are presented in **Table 2**, with an indication of the CT ID.

3.1. Monoclonal antibodies (mAbs)

One of the most intensively explored passive immunotherapeutic approach resorts to mAbs. These are able to recognize cell surface receptors and ligands, which provide a successful strategy to target antigens highly expressed in tumor cells or receptors involved in tumorigenesis [6]. They can function through a set of ways, such as by blocking ligand-receptor binding and/or downstream signaling pathways, targeting the tumor microenvironment, immune cells or immunosuppressive tumor microenvironments, and modulating constant fragment (Fc) domain of antibodies [48].

The mAbs have been applied as immunotherapeutic agents in GBM treatment. Two targets expressed on GBM cells are vascular endothelial growth factor (VEGF) and EGFR or its variant III mutation EGFRvIII. Bevacizumab, a humanized antibody against VEGF, was the first mAb studied in the treatment of GBM patients. This mAb has the ability to promote the blockade of VEGF pathway, intervening in neovascularization of the tumor and, consequently, in tumor growth, decreasing its size [49, 50]. It was approved by the food and drug administration (FDA) in 2009 for recurrent GBM. Two phase II multicenter and randomized CT were performed to evaluate the safety of bevacizumab with or without irinotecan (a cytotoxic prodrug which inhibits DNA replication and activates apoptotic cell death) in patients with recurrent GBM, where treatment-associated toxicity was documented in some of the patients [51]. For newly diagnosed GBM patients, this drug has been investigated together with standard therapy in comparative studies to assess the use of bevacizumab as first-line treatment. Two randomized double-blind placebo-control trials [52, 53] and one open-label single-arm phase II CT [54] showed that the addition of bevacizumab to standard therapy prolonged the progression-free survival (PFS), but did not improve OS. Additionally, serious adverse events related to bevacizumab were also reported in these trials. Thus, the efficacy of bevacizumab on quality of life of newly diagnosed GBM patients was not clearly specified and further well-designed CT should be performed. Other ongoing CT of bevacizumab agent in GBM treatment are present in **Table 2**. Inversely to bevacizumab, there are other mAbs agents that specifically target EGFR and/or EGFRvIII, which are the most common tumor-expressed targets explored in antibody therapy. EGFR is expressed in approximately 40% of GBM patients and 65% of them present EGFRvIII mutation [49]. These mAbs have the ability to blockade ligand binding or signaling through these receptors, interfering with tumor growth rates and inducing

Strategy	Drug/antigen	Other therapy	Clinical phase (status)	Clinical trial ID
mAbs	Bevacizumab	–	I/II (recruiting)	NCT01811498
		–	II (not recruiting)	NCT02157103
		TMZ	III (recruiting)	NCT02761070
		TMZ	II (not recruiting)	NCT01149850
	Nimotuzumab	RT plus TMZ	III (completed)	NCT00753246
		RT plus TMZ	II (completed)	NCT03388372
	Cetuximab	RT plus TMZ	I/II (recruiting)	NCT02861898
	ABT-414	RT plus TMZ	I (completed)	NCT01800695
		RT plus TMZ	III (recruiting)	NCT02573324
		TMZ or lomustine	II (recruiting)	NCT02343406
	AMG595	–	I (completed)	NCT01475006
Immune checkpoint inhibitors	Nivolumab (anti-PD-1)	RT and TMZ	III (recruiting)	NCT02617589
		RT plus TMZ	III (recruiting)	NCT02667587
	Pembrolizumab (anti-PD-L1)	–	Pilot (recruiting)	NCT02852655
		RT plus TMZ	I/II (not recruiting)	NCT02530502
		Bevacizumab	II (not recruiting)	NCT02337491
		RT plus TMZ; HSPPC-96 vaccine	II (recruiting)	NCT03018288
	Durvalumab (anti-PD-L1)	Bevacizumab or RT	II (not recruiting)	NCT02336165
	Avelumab (anti-PD-L1)	RT plus TMZ	II (recruiting)	NCT03047473
	Nivolumab (anti-PD-1) and ipilimumab (anti-CTLA-4)	TMZ	I (not recruiting)	NCT02311920
		Bevacizumab	III (not recruiting)	NCT02017717
Adoptive T-cell therapy	CMV-CTL	TMZ	I/II (recruiting)	NCT02661282
	CMV-ALT	RT plus TMZ	I (completed)	NCT00693095
CAR T-cell therapy	IL-13Rα2	–	I (recruiting)	NCT02208362
		–	Pilot (completed)	NCT00730613
	EphA2	–	I/II (completed)	NCT02575261
	HER2	CMV-CTL	I (not recruiting)	NCT01109095
		–	I/II (recruiting)	NCT02713984
		RT plus TMZ	I (recruiting)	NCT02442297
	EGFRvIII	Fludarabine and cyclophosphamide	Pilot (recruiting)	NCT02844062
		Fludarabine, cyclophosphamide and IL-2	I/II (recruiting)	NCT01454596
		–	I (not recruiting)	NCT02209376
		RT plus TMZ	I (recruiting)	NCT02664363

Strategy	Drug/antigen	Other therapy	Clinical phase (status)	Clinical trial ID
OVs	HSV-1 M032	—	I (recruiting)	NCT02062827
	DNX-2401	TMZ	I (completed)	NCT01956734
		IFN-γ	I (not recruiting)	NCT02197169
		—	I (recruiting)	NCT03178032
		Pembrolizumab	II (recruiting)	NCT02798406
	AdV-tK	RT and valacyclovir	II (completed)	NCT00589875
		RT and valacyclovir	I (completed)	NCT00751270
	Reolysin	RT and/or chemotherapy	I (completed)	NCT00528684

mAbs: monoclonal antibodies; TMZ: temozolomide; RT: radiotherapy; PD-1: programmed cell death protein 1; CTLA-4: cytotoxic T-lymphocyte-associated protein 4; HSPPC-96: heat-shock protein peptide complex 96; CMV-CTL: cytomegalovirus cytotoxic T lymphocytes; CMV-ALT: cytomegalovirus autologous lymphocyte transfer; CAR: chimeric antigen receptor; IL-13Rα2: interleukin-13 receptor alpha 2; HER2: human epidermal growth factor receptor 2; EphA2: erythropoietin-producing hepatocellular carcinoma 2; EGFRvIII: epidermal growth factor receptor variant III mutation; IL-2: interleukin-2; Ovs: oncolytic viruses; HSV: herpes simplex virus (HSV); IFN-γ: interferon gamma; AdV-tK: adenovirus mutant thymidine kinase.

Table 2. Representative CT of immunotherapeutic strategies in GBM treatment, including mAbs, immune checkpoint inhibitors, adoptive T-cell therapy, CAR T-cell therapy and OVs.

apoptosis, as well as providing a better sensitization of tumors to chemotherapeutic agents [48]. Examples of these mAbs are nimotuzumab and cetuximab, which are tested in clinical stage with early promising outcomes in the majority of the cases. More details about their CT are displayed in **Table 2**.

A recent and promising strategy using mAbs is based on antibody drug-conjugate (ADC), where mAbs are linked to cytotoxic molecules that specifically target tumor cells, promoting delivery of drugs or toxins. ABT-414 and AMG595 are two examples of ADCs that specifically target EGFRvIII and are under investigation for the treatment of GBM (**Table 2**) [49, 50].

3.2. Immune checkpoint inhibitors

Immune checkpoints are molecules that can attenuate the strength and duration of the normal activity of CTLs and are responsible for preventing autoimmunity and mitigating collateral tissue damage [5, 55, 56]. Programmed cell death protein 1 (PD-1) and cytotoxic T-lymphocyte-associated protein 4 (CTLA-4) is the most studied immune checkpoints molecules that provide immune resistance mechanisms at different levels and by different mechanisms, leading to inhibition of T-cell proliferation and cytokine production, consequently resulting in a non-activation of T-cells [2, 56]. Both PD-1 and CTLA-4 are receptors expressed on the surface of T-cells [51]. PD-1 blocks T-cells at advanced stages of the immune response and interact with one of the PD-1 ligands expressed on the surface of tumor cells (such as PD-L1/B7.H1 or PD-L2/B7-DC), while CTLA-4 occurs early in T-cell immune response and binds to ligands expressed on the surface of APCs (such as B7.1/CD80 and B7.2/CD86) [2, 56].

A strategy based on the blockade of these inhibitory receptors and their ligands through the use of antibodies has been explored as a promising immunotherapeutic approach for diverse solid tumors, such as glioblastoma, inducing T-cell-mediated antitumor immunity [6]. PD-1 is expressed on activated T-cells, B-cells, DCs and macrophages and the expression of PD-L1 has been reported in glioma cell lines and tumor tissues, as well as in activated APCs in glioma patients, and its level of occurrence is associated with glioma grade [55]. Preclinical studies using antibodies to target PD-1/PD-L1 in animal glioma models showed encouraging results, especially in combination with radiotherapy [2, 57], which provided a strong support to proceed to clinical stage. Several CT are ongoing to evaluate the safety and efficacy of anti-PD-1/PD-L1 human antibodies, namely nivolumab (anti-PD-1 antibody) and pembrolizumab (anti-PD-L1 antibody), which have been tested alone or in combination with other agents in GBM patients. Some of these trials are in early phases, but two phase III trials are evaluating nivolumab and comparing it with standard therapy (NCT02617589 and NCT02667587). In a preclinical stage, the anti-CTLA-4 strategy has also demonstrated robust and effective response rates, with an increasing of long-term survival in 80% of treated mice [5]. Clinically, the safety and efficacy of nivolumab with or without ipilumumab, an anti-CTLA-4 human antibody, in GBM patients, are assessed in phase I and III trials (NCT02311920 and NCT02017717, respectively). This combinatorial PD-1 and CTLA-4 blockade demonstrated the most effective results. More information about immune checkpoint inhibitors trials is summarized in **Table 2**.

Despite their great impact on survival, this immunotherapeutic approach presents some limitations, reflected by the immune-associated side effects experienced by some patients, such as dermatological, endocrinological, gastrointestinal, and hepatic toxicities, which have been reported like associated with the abnormal infiltration of stimulated CD4+–CD8+ T-cells into normal tissues with the concurrent elevation of levels of pro-inflammatory cytokines [2].

3.3. Chimeric antigen receptor (CAR) T-cell therapy

Adoptive T-cell therapy has also been widely applied in treatment of highly aggressive and advanced tumors, including GBM [58]. This therapy is based on direct T-cells activation and can be described in a simple way through the isolation of tumor-specific autologous T-cells and *in vitro* expansion followed by their injection into the patient, in order to improve antitumor activity [5, 6]. As referred previously, CMV has been suggested as a potential GBM therapeutic target, due to the expression of its antigens in GBM cells, but not in surrounding healthy brain tissue. In a phase I CT for recurrent GBM patients, the feasibility and safety of a combinatorial therapy of autologous adoptively CMV-specific T-cell therapy and chemotherapy were demonstrated, highlighting the power of this antiviral therapy to improve GBM prognosis [59]. Other examples of CTs regarding CMV adoptive T-cell therapy are depicted in **Table 2**. However, it has been observed that this immunotherapeutic strategy is limited by the immunosuppressive tumor microenvironment, and the need of T-cells to recognize tumor antigens presented by the MHC class I [2, 60].

A novel type of adoptive T-cell therapy that has been proposed to overcome these shortcomings, is based on the transference of autologous T-cells genetically modified with CARs [5]. CARs are cell surface receptors selected to establish a high specificity with tumor cells and provide T-cell activation through a mechanism where the antigen-binding region of a mAb is fused with the T-cell receptor (TCR) signaling domain CD3. They allow an antibody-like antigen recognition in a non-MHC-restricted pathway and a more effective T-cell penetration and persistence into the tumor microenvironment than mAbs [60, 61]. The implementation of CAR T-cell therapy in GBM treatment has demonstrated to be highly promising, where several GBM-specific antigens have been investigated as targets, such as (IL-13Rα2), human epidermal growth factor receptor 2 (HER2), erythropoietin-producing hepatocellular carcinoma 2 (EphA2) and EGFRvIII [50, 61]. Preclinical studies that involve these targets are associated with positive outcomes, and all of them are also ongoing in a clinical stage [5]. A pilot study of intracranial delivery of CAR T-cells targeting IL-13Rα2 into the resection cavity of three patients with recurrent GBM (NCT00730613) provided preliminary results about its safety and feasibility, showing that the strategy was well-tolerated without the emergence of serious side effects. Further, a transient antitumor activity was developed in two of the patients and the decrease of IL-13Rα2 expression within the tumor was confirmed in one patient [62]. Regarding the application of CAR T-cells therapy for EphA2 positive malignant glioma patients, a phase I/II CT (NCT02575261) was completed, where the effectiveness, safety, and clinical response were evaluated, but the results have not yet been published. A phase I trial of CMV-specific CAR T-cells therapy targeting HER2 (NCT01109095), considered a more active strategy that reacts with the virus and tumor cells is also in progress to investigate its safety and efficacy in the treatment of patients with GBM. Several clinical trials exploring CAR T-cells targeting EGFRvIII in GBM are underway to test the safety and effectiveness of this approach. More detailed information about these CAR T-cell clinical trials, as well as other examples, can be found in **Table 2**. Phase I/II clinical trials have provided early results of potential efficacy with an acceptable toxicity profile, but more efforts need to be carried out to assess the efficacy of the application of CAR T-cell therapy in GBM treatment. Despite the tolerable toxicity, cytokine release syndrome (CRS) is the most frequent adverse effect due to the extreme immune activation, especially evidenced in the case of intravenous administration. Furthermore, additional disadvantages are the high cost of the therapy and the possibility of expression of the target antigen on healthy tissues [61].

3.4. Oncolytic viruses (OVs)

Oncolytic virotherapy is another emerging immunotherapeutic strategy that has been investigated in the treatment of GBM, evidencing promising results. OVs are replication-competent viral vectors used to induce effective antiviral and antitumor immune responses [2, 51]. They are able to selectively replicate in tumor cells through cell surface marker identification, induce tumor cell death, spread within the tumor and indirectly recruit immune cells to promote immune responses against themselves and infected and uninfected tumor cells [58, 63]. They can naturally occur or are genetically manipulated to specifically infect and destroy tumor cells overexpressing tumor antigens [50, 51]. Once all the tumor cells are eradicated, the excess of virus can be removed using an anti-viral medication [49]. Several OVs are under investigation for GBM targeting. Some of them have been tested at different stages of CTs, including herpes simplex virus (HSV), adenovirus (AdV), measles virus (MV), poliovirus (PV), reovirus, H1 parvovirus and Newcastle disease virus (NDV), after preclinical researches showing antitumor activity, and many of the remaining OVs are in advanced preclinical stages [63].

HSV is a neurotropic human pathogen that provides tumor selectivity with safety and the most intensively studied examples of genetically modified mutant HSV are G207 and HSV1716 [51]. Phase I and Ib trials performed to evaluate the safety of G207 inoculation into the brain resection cavity for recurrent GBM showed no treatment-related toxicity neither serious adverse effects, with no patients developing HSV encephalitis, and encouraging therapeutic efficacy was reported [2]. Another phase I trial that combines G207 oncolytic HSV therapy with radiotherapy also demonstrated safety and potential antitumor activity in the treatment of recurrent GBM patients [64]. HSV1716 is also reported in phase I trials, where no toxicity ascribed to HSV1716 was demonstrated [65, 66]. Another example of a genetically modified mutant HSV that has been investigated (HSV-1 M032) is presented in **Table 2**. Relatively to genetically engineered AdVs, which are non-enveloped virus with a double-stranded linear DNA genome, the most commonly investigated in GBM treatment are DNX-2401, ONYX-015 and AdV-tK [2, 49–51]. In the case of DNX-2401, the tumor targeting is achieved and increased due to the presence of cyclic arginine/glycine/aspartic acid (cRGD) peptide that permits the attachment to host's immune cells [50]. In a phase I trial of DNX-2401 oncolytic AdV, patients with recurrent high-grade glioma were subjected to an intratumoral injection in a dose escalation, demonstrating that this AdV is able to infect, replicate in and kill human glioma cells, without a harming toxicity profile. Furthermore, despite the early stage of the trial, a promising efficacy was expected, where 12% of the patients demonstrate durable complete therapeutic responses [67]. Other phase I CTs of DNX-2401 are displayed in **Table 2**. On the other hand, ONYX-015 oncolytic AdV was also tested in a phase I trial, through intracerebral injection of various doses in patients with recurrent glioma that was resected, where no serious related-treatment adverse events were identified, even at the highest administered dose [2]. For AdV-tK, an AdV mutant thymidine kinase, a randomized phase II trial (NCT00870181) was carried out with the parallel administration of ganciclovir, showing an improvement of PFS and OS in the treatment of patients with recurrent high grade glioma. Other CTs of AdV-tK are presented in **Table 2**. MV is an RNA virus and the genetically modified derivatives of MVs, such as modified Edmonston (MV-Edm) vaccine, have an affinity for cellular CD46 receptor abundantly expressed on tumor cells [2]. In addition, with the aim of facilitating *in vivo* monitoring of viral gene expression and replication, this MV has been engineered to express the human carcinoembryonic antigen (CEA; MV-Edm-CEA), which is expressed by various types of cancers, but not by gliomas [51]. However, MV-Edm-CEA has exhibited a great potential as an oncolytic therapy for GBM in preclinical studies. A phase I CTs with this MV (NCT00390299) was initiated to evaluate the MV-Edm-CEA-associated adverse effects and its best dose in patients with recurrent GBM, however, this study was recently suspended by reasons not yet reported. PV is an enterovirus that encompasses a protein capsid and RNA, expressing high-affinity for neoplastic cells and tropism to motor neurons [51]. A genetically recombinant polio/rhinovirus chimera, PVSRIPO, was developed to reduce the neurotoxicity frequently observed in cases of human poliomyelitis, avoiding neuvirulence tendency. This PV recognize the CD155 cell surface polio receptor, a tumor antigen widely expressed in tumor cells, including GBM [51, 58]. A phase I trial is underway to evaluate the safety and the occurrence of potential antitumor responses of intratumoral administration of PVSRIPO in patients with recurrent GBM (NCT01491893). Preliminary reported results of this clinical trial described that the infusion of PVSRIPO was well-tolerated and revealed a promising efficacy, as well as provided a survival advantage when compared to historical control group of patients that was also analyzed [51]. Reovirus is a double-stranded RNA virus that is isolated from the respiratory and gastrointestinal tracts of humans. The safety of intratumoral administration in a dose-escalation of this genetically unmodified OV was also assessed in a phase I trial in patients with recurrent GBM that received prior radiotherapy with or without chemotherapy [68]. More information about a phase I trial of reolysin, a genetically engineered reovirus, is depicted in **Table 2**.

The use of OVs has been shown through some CTs as a harmless strategy with promising results; however, no OV has yet been approved by the FDA for GBM [58]. On the other hand, their therapeutic efficacy needs to be thoroughly assessed and proven with convincing clinical success in advanced phase trials. This task is hampered by the high genetic heterogeneity of GBM, and the ability of BBB to inhibit migration of OVs to the tumor site, thus compromising the success of the treatment [6].

4. Conclusions

The current, first line, GBM standard therapy has not provided the necessary and expected improvements in overall patient survival rates. Immunotherapy is being explored as an alternative strategy, revealing to be a promising field, associated with good outcomes and fewer adverse events.

The advances in technology, as well as in scientific knowledge regarding gene expression and signaling pathways analysis, have provided data to translate into new perspectives on personalized therapeutic approaches. In this context, immunotherapy has gained importance insofar as the identification of specific biomarkers in each patient could be useful for prognosis of personal immune responses. Several immunotherapeutic CTs are currently ongoing for GBM, predominantly using vaccines, and the preliminary results attained so far yielded satisfactory clinical responses associated with antitumor activity. However, some challenges have been reported, which are associated to finding therapeutic agents capable to penetrate the BBB, the identification of suitable, specific and immunogenic tumor antigens and appropriate pre- and post-therapeutic markers in order to develop immune-targeted agents. Other limitations comprise the reduced number of GBM patients skilled to incorporate particular clinical studies, and the insufficient understanding of the immune system as well as the GBM microenvironment. Given the molecular heterogeneity and immunosuppression that so well depict the GBM, combinatorial therapies targeting multiple pathways now become a need and so they have already been explored. A variety of regimens have been equated, combining immunotherapeutic strategies (vaccines, cell therapies, multiple checkpoint inhibitors, and antibodies) along with molecules targeting either tumor cells or their microenvironment, as well the current standard therapy. Consequently, more advanced CTs need to be underway to deeply explore the fundamental insights of these therapies. In addition, the discovery of new targets and mechanisms is essential in order to help widespread this field of research, and develop optimized therapeutic strategies for GBM.

Acknowledgements

This paper was supported by the Fundação para a Ciência e a Tecnologia (FCT), Portuguese Agency for Scientific Research, through: the project no. 016648 (Ref. POCI-01-0145-FEDER-016648), the project PEst-UID/NEU/04539/2013, and COMPETE (Ref. POCI-01-0145-FEDER-007440) - Centre for Neurosciences and Cell Biology (CNC); the projects PEst-OE/QUI/UI0313/2014 and POCI-01-0145-FEDER-007630 - Coimbra Chemistry Centre; and the project UID/QUI/50006/2013 - LAQV/REQUIMTE.

Conflict of interest

The authors declare they have no conflict of interest.

Author details

Jessica Silva[1,2†], Ana Miranda[1,2†], João Sousa[1,3], Alberto Pais[4*] and Carla Vitorino[1,2,3]

*Address all correspondence to: pais@qui.uc.pt

1 Faculty of Pharmacy, University of Coimbra, Coimbra, Portugal

2 Centre for Neurosciences and Cell Biology (CNC), University of Coimbra, Coimbra, Portugal

3 Laqv Requimte, Group of Pharmaceutical Technology, Porto, Portugal

4 Coimbra Chemistry Center, Department of Chemistry, University of Coimbra, Coimbra, Portugal

† These authors contributed equally to this work and should be regarded as co-first authors.

References

[1] Alifieris C, Trafalis DT. Glioblastoma multiforme: Pathogenesis and treatment. Pharmacology & Therapeutics. 2015;**152**:63-82. DOI: 10.1016/j.pharmthera.2015.05.005

[2] Calinescu A-A, Kamran N, Baker G, Mineharu Y, Lowenstein PR, Castro MG. Overview of current immunotherapeutic strategies for glioma. Immunotherapy. 2015;**7**(10):1073-1104. DOI: 10.2217/imt.15.75

[3] Louis DN, Ohgaki H, Wiestler OD, Cavenee WK. WHO Classification of Tumours of the Central Nervous System. Lyon: International Agency for Research on Cancer; 2016

[4] Chen PY, Wei KC, Liu HL. Neural immune modulation and immunotherapy assisted by focused ultrasound induced blood-brain barrier opening. Human Vaccines & Immunotherapeutics. 2015;**11**(11):2682-2687. DOI: 10.1080/21645515.2015.1071749

[5] Huang B, Zhang H, Gu L, Ye B, Jian Z, Stary C, et al. Advances in immunotherapy for glioblastoma multiforme. Journal of Immunology Research. 2017;**2017**:3597613. DOI: 10.1155/2017/3597613

[6] Lyon JG, Mokarram N, Saxena T, Carroll SL, Bellamkonda RV. Engineering challenges for brain tumor immunotherapy. Advanced Drug Delivery Reviews. 2017;**114**:19-32. DOI: 10.1016/j.addr.2017.06.006

[7] Xu LW, Chow KKH, Lim M, Li G. Current vaccine trials in glioblastoma: A review. Journal of Immunology Research. 2014;**2014**:10. DOI: 10.1155/2014/796856

[8] Bilusic M, Madan RA. Therapeutic cancer vaccines: The latest advancement in targeted therapy. American Journal of Therapeutics. 2012;**19**(6):e172-e181. DOI: 10.1097/MJT.0b013e3182068cdb

[9] Kalinski P, Urban J, Narang R, Berk E, Wieckowski E, Muthuswamy R. Dendritic cell-based therapeutic cancer vaccines: What we have and what we need. Future Oncology. 2009;**5**(3):379-390. DOI: 10.2217/fon.09.6

[10] Butterfield LH. Cancer vaccines. BMJ. 2015;**350**:h988. DOI: 10.1136/bmj.h988

[11] Srinivasan VM, Ferguson SD, Lee S, Weathers SP, Kerrigan BCP, Heimberger AB. Tumor vaccines for malignant gliomas. Neurotherapeutics. 2017;**14**(2):345-357. DOI: 10.1007/s13311-017-0522-2

[12] Kurtz SL, Ravindranathan S, Zaharoff DA. Current status of autologous breast tumor cell-based vaccines. Expert Review of Vaccines. 2014;**13**(12):1439-1445. DOI: 10.1586/14760584.2014.969714

[13] Yamaguchi Y, Yamaue H, Okusaka T, Okuno K, Suzuki H, Fujioka T, et al. Guidance for peptide vaccines for the treatment of cancer. Cancer Science. 2014;**105**(7):924-931. DOI: 10.1111/cas.12443

[14] Sampson JH, Mitchell DA. Vaccination strategies for neuro-oncology. Neuro-Oncology. 2015;**17**(Suppl 7):vii15-vii25. DOI: 10.1093/neuonc/nov159

[15] Swartz AM, Batich KA, Fecci PE, Sampson JH. Peptide vaccines for the treatment of glioblastoma. Journal of Neuro-Oncology. 2015;**123**(3):433-440. DOI: 10.1007/s11060-014-1676-y

[16] Slingluff CL. The present and future of peptide vaccines for cancer: Single or multiple, long or short, alone or in combination? Cancer Journal. 2011;**17**(5):343-350. DOI: 10.1097/PPO.0b013e318233e5b2

[17] Elsamadicy AA, Chongsathidkiet P, Desai R, Woroniecka K, Farber SH, Fecci PE, et al. Prospect of rindopepimut in the treatment of glioblastoma. Expert Opinion on Biological Therapy. 2017;**17**(4):507-513. DOI: 10.1080/14712598.2017.1299705

[18] Winograd EK, Ciesielski MJ, Fenstermaker RA. Novel vaccines for glioblastoma: Clinical update and perspective. Immunotherapy. 2016;**8**(11):1293-1308. DOI: 10.2217/imt-2016-0059

[19] Fenstermaker RA, Ciesielski MJ, Qiu J, Yang N, Frank CL, Lee KP, et al. Clinical study of a survivin long peptide vaccine (SurVaxM) in patients with recurrent malignant glioma. Cancer Immunology, Immunotherapy. 2016;**65**(11):1339-1352. DOI: 10.1007/s00262-016-1890-x

[20] Kamran N, Calinescu A, Candolfi M, Chandran M, Mineharu Y, Assad AS, et al. Recent advances and future of immunotherapy for glioblastoma. Expert Opinion on Biological Therapy. 2016;**16**(10):1245-1264. DOI: 10.1080/14712598.2016.1212012

[21] Chianese-Bullock KA, Lewis ST, Sherman NE, Shannon JD, Slingluff CL. Multi-peptide vaccines vialed as peptide mixtures can be stable reagents for use in peptide-based immune therapies. Vaccine. 2009;**27**(11):1764-1770. DOI: 10.1016/j.vaccine.2009.01.018

[22] Binabaj MM, Bahrami A, ShahidSales S, Joodi M, Joudi Mashhad M, Hassanian SM. The prognostic value of MGMT promoter methylation in glioblastoma: A meta-analysis of clinical trials. Journal of Cellular Physiology. 2018;**233**(1):378-386. DOI: 10.1002/jcp.25896

[23] Chatterjee S, Burns TF. Targeting heat shock proteins in cancer: A promising therapeutic approach. International Journal of Molecular Sciences. 2017;**18**(9). DOI: 10.3390/ijms18091978

[24] Graner MW, Bigner DD. Chaperone proteins and brain tumors: Potential targets and possible therapeutics. Neuro-Oncology. 2005;**7**(3):260-277. DOI: 10.1215/S1152851704001188

[25] Ampie L, Choy W, Lamano JB, Fakurnejad S, Bloch O, Parsa AT. Heat shock protein vaccines against glioblastoma: From bench to bedside. Journal of Neuro-Oncology. 2015;**123**(3):441-448. DOI: 10.1007/s11060-015-1837-7

[26] Ampie L, Choy W, Lamano JB, Fakurnejad S, Bloch O, Parsa AT. Heatshock protein vaccines against glioblastoma: From bench to bedside. Journal of Neuro-Oncology. 2015;**123**(3):441-448. DOI: 10.1007/s11060-015-1837-7

[27] Lee C, Lee M, Rhee I. Distinct features of dendritic cell-based immunotherapy as cancer vaccines. Clinical and Experimental Vaccine Research. 2018;**7**(1):16-23. DOI: 10.7774/cevr.2018.7.1.16

[28] Janikashvili N, Larmonier N, Katsanis E. Personalized dendritic cell-based tumor immunotherapy. Immunotherapy. 2010;**2**(1):57. DOI: 10.2217/imt.09.78

[29] Elster JD, Krishnadas DK, Lucas KG. Dendritic cell vaccines: A review of recent developments and their potential pediatric application. Human Vaccines & Immunotherapeutics. 2016;**12**(9):2232-2239. DOI: 10.1080/21645515.2016.1179844

[30] Lathia JD, Mack SC, Mulkearns-Hubert EE, Valentim CLL, Rich JN. Cancer stem cells in glioblastoma. Genes & Development. 2015;**29**(12):1203-1217. DOI: 10.1101/gad.261982.115

[31] Vik-Mo EO, Nyakas M, Mikkelsen BV, Moe MC, Due-Tønnesen P, Suso EMI, et al. Therapeutic vaccination against autologous cancer stem cells with mRNA-transfected dendritic cells in patients with glioblastoma. Cancer Immunology, Immunotherapy. 2013;**62**(9):1499-1509. DOI: 10.1007/s00262-013-1453-3

[32] Dunn-Pirio A, Peters K, DesJardins A, Randazzo D, Friedman H, Healy P, et al. Tumor stem cell RNA-loaded dendritic cell vaccine for recurrent glioblastoma: A phase 1 trial (S41.004). Neurology. 2017;**88**(16 Supplement)

[33] Rainone V, Martelli C, Ottobrini L, Biasin M, Borelli M, Lucignani G, et al. Immunological characterization of whole tumour lysate-loaded dendritic cells for cancer immunotherapy. PLoS One. 2016;**11**(1):e0146622. DOI: 10.1371/journal.pone.0146622

[34] Hdeib A, Sloan AE. Dendritic cell immunotherapy for solid tumors: Evaluation of the DCVax(R) platform in the treatment of glioblastoma multiforme. CNS Oncology. 2015;**4**(2):63-69. DOI: 10.2217/cns.14.54

[35] Nair SK, De Leon G, Boczkowski D, Schmittling R, Xie W, Staats J, et al. Recognition and killing of autologous, primary glioblastoma tumor cells by human cytomegalovirus pp65-specific cytotoxic T cells. Clinical Cancer Research. 2014;**20**(10):2684-2694. DOI: 10.1158/1078-0432.ccr-13-3268

[36] Tanaka M, Tsuno NH, Fujii T, Todo T, Saito N, Takahashi K. Human umbilical vein endothelial cell vaccine therapy in patients with recurrent glioblastoma. Cancer Science. 2013;**104**(2):200-205. DOI: 10.1111/cas.12055

[37] Sakamoto N, Uemae Y, Ishikawa E, Takano S, Nakai K, Yamamoto T, et al. Glioma immunotherapy with combined autologous tumor cell and endothelial cell vaccine in vivo. Neurologia Medico-Chirurgica (Tokyo). 2012;**52**(4):194-201. DOI: 10.2176/nmc.52.194

[38] Okaji Y, Tsuno NH, Tanaka M, Yoneyama S, Matsuhashi M, Kitayama J, et al. Pilot study of anti-angiogenic vaccine using fixed whole endothelium in patients with progressive malignancy after failure of conventional therapy. European Journal of Cancer. 2008;**44**(3):383-390. DOI: 10.1016/j.ejca.2007.10.018

[39] Ishikawa E, Muragaki Y, Yamamoto T, Maruyama T, Tsuboi K, Ikuta S, et al. Phase I/IIa trial of fractionated radiotherapy, temozolomide, and autologous formalin-fixed tumor vaccine for newly diagnosed glioblastoma. Journal of Neurosurgery. 2014;**121**(3):543-553. DOI: 10.3171/2014.5.jns132392

[40] Ishikawa E, Tsuboi K, Yamamoto T, Muroi A, Takano S, Enomoto T, et al. Clinical trial of autologous formalin-fixed tumor vaccine for glioblastoma multiforme patients. Cancer Science. 2007;**98**(8):1226-1233. DOI: 10.1111/j.1349-7006.2007.00518.x

[41] Kumai T, Kobayashi H, Harabuchi Y, Celis E. Peptide vaccines in cancer-old concept revisited. Current Opinion in Immunology. 2017;**45**:1-7. DOI: 10.1016/j.coi.2016.11.001

[42] Itoh K, Yamada A. Personalized peptide vaccines: A new therapeutic modality for cancer. Cancer Science. 2006;**97**(10):970-976. DOI: 10.1111/j.1349-7006.2006.00272.x

[43] Datta J, Terhune JH, Lowenfeld L, Cintolo JA, Xu S, Roses RE, et al. Optimizing dendritic cell-based approaches for cancer immunotherapy. The Yale Journal of Biology and Medicine. 2014;**87**(4):491-518

[44] Cintolo JA, Datta J, Mathew SJ, Czerniecki BJ. Dendritic cell-based vaccines: Barriers and opportunities. Future Oncology. 2012;**8**(10):1273-1299. DOI: 10.2217/fon.12.125

[45] Keenan BP, Jaffee EM. Whole cell vaccines--past progress and future strategies. Seminars in Oncology. 2012;**39**(3):276-286. DOI: 10.1053/j.seminoncol.2012.02.007

[46] Copier J, Dalgleish A. Overview of tumor cell-based vaccines. International Reviews of Immunology. 2006;**25**(5-6):297-319. DOI: 10.1080/08830180600992472

[47] ClinicalTrials.gov [12-03-2018]. Available from: https://clinicaltrials.gov/ct2/home

[48] Weiner LM, Surana R, Wang S. Monoclonal antibodies: Versatile platforms for cancer immunotherapy. Nature Reviews. Immunology. 2010;**10**(5):317-327. DOI: 10.1038/nri2744

[49] Carlsson SK, Brothers SP, Wahlestedt C. Emerging treatment strategies for glioblastoma multiforme. EMBO Molecular Medicine. 2014;**6**(11):1359-1370. DOI: 10.15252/emmm.201302627

[50] Paolillo M, Boselli C, Schinelli S. Glioblastoma under siege: An overview of current therapeutic strategies. Brain Sciences. 2018;**8**(1):pii: E15. DOI: 10.3390/brainsci8010015

[51] Dunn-Pirio AM, Vlahovic G. Immunotherapy approaches in the treatment of malignant brain tumors. Cancer. 2017;**123**(5):734-750. DOI: 10.1002/cncr.30371

[52] Gilbert MR, Dignam JJ, Armstrong TS, Wefel JS, Blumenthal DT, Vogelbaum MA, et al. A randomized trial of bevacizumab for newly diagnosed glioblastoma. The New England Journal of Medicine. 2014;**370**(8):699-708. DOI: 10.1056/NEJMoa1308573

[53] Chinot OL, Wick W, Mason W, Henriksson R, Saran F, Nishikawa R, et al. Bevacizumab plus radiotherapy–temozolomide for newly diagnosed glioblastoma. The New England Journal of Medicine. 2014;**370**(8):709-722. DOI: 10.1056/NEJMoa1308345

[54] Lai A, Tran A, Nghiemphu PL, Pope WB, Solis OE, Selch M, et al. Phase II study of bevacizumab plus temozolomide during and after radiation therapy for patients with newly diagnosed glioblastoma multiforme. Journal of Clinical Oncology. 2011;**29**(2):142-148. DOI: 10.1200/JCO.2010.30.2729

[55] Xue S, Hu M, Iyer V. Yu J. Blocking the PD-1/PD-L1 pathway in glioma: A potential new treatment strategy. Journal of Hematology & Oncology. 2017;**10**(1):81. DOI: 10.1186/s13045-017-0455-6

[56] Pardoll DM. The blockade of immune checkpoints in cancer immunotherapy. Nature Reviews Cancer. 2012;**12**(4):252-264. DOI: 10.1038/nrc3239

[57] Xue S, Hu M, Li P, Ma J, Xie L, Teng F, et al. Relationship between expression of PD-L1 and tumor angiogenesis, proliferation, and invasion in glioma. Oncotarget. 2017;**8**(30):49702-49712. DOI: 10.18632/oncotarget.17922

[58] Desai R, Suryadevara CM, Batich KA, Farber SH, Sanchez-Perez L, Sampson JH. Emerging immunotherapies for glioblastoma. Expert Opinion on Emerging Drugs. 2016;**21**(2):133-145. DOI: 10.1080/14728214.2016.1186643

[59] Schuessler A, Smith C, Beagley L, Boyle GM, Rehan S, Matthews K, et al. Autologous T-cell therapy for cytomegalovirus as a consolidative treatment for recurrent glioblastoma. Cancer Research. 2014;**74**(13):3466-3476. DOI: 10.1158/0008-5472.CAN-14-0296

[60] Bielamowicz KJ, Khawja S, Ahmed N. Adoptive cell therapies for glioblastoma. Frontiers in Oncology. 2013;**3**:275. DOI: 10.3389/fonc.2013.00275

[61] Rodriguez A, Brown C, Badie B. Chimeric antigen receptor T-cell therapy for glioblastoma. Translational Research. 2017;**187**:93-102. DOI: 10.4049/jimmunol.1701155

[62] Brown CE, Badie B, Barish ME, Weng L, Ostberg JR, Chang W-C, et al. Bioactivity and safety of IL13Rα2-redirected chimeric antigen receptor CD8+ T cells in patients with recurrent glioblastoma. Clinical Cancer Research. 2015;**21**(18):4062-4072. DOI: 10.1158/1078-0432.CCR-15-0428

[63] Wollmann G, Ozduman K, van den Pol AN. Oncolytic virus therapy of glioblastoma multiforme–concepts and candidates. Cancer Journal. 2012;**18**(1):69-81. DOI: 10.1097/PPO.0b013e31824671c9

[64] Markert JM, Razdan SN, Kuo H-C, Cantor A, Knoll A, Karrasch M, et al. A phase 1 trial of oncolytic HSV-1, G207, given in combination with radiation for recurrent GBM demonstrates safety and radiographic responses. Molecular Therapy. 2014;**22**(5):1048-1055. DOI: 10.1038/mt.2014.22

[65] Papanastassiou V, Rampling R, Fraser M, Petty R, Hadley D, Nicoll J, et al. The potential for efficacy of the modified (ICP 34.5–) herpes simplex virus HSV1716 following intratumoural injection into human malignant glioma: A proof of principle study. Gene Therapy. 2002;**9**(6):398-406. DOI: 10.1038/sj.gt.3301664

[66] Kambara H, Okano H, Chiocca EA, Saeki Y. An oncolytic HSV-1 mutant expressing ICP34. 5 under control of a nestin promoter increases survival of animals even when symptomatic from a brain tumor. Cancer Research. 2005;**65**(7):2832-2839. DOI: 10.1158/0008-5472.CAN-04-3227

[67] Lang FF, Conrad C, Gomez-Manzano C, Tufaro F, Yung W, Sawaya R, et al. First-in-human phase I clinical trial of oncolytic delta-24-rgd (dnx-2401) with biological endpoints: Implications for viro-immunotherapy. Neuro-Oncology. 2014;**16**(Suppl 3):iii39. DOI: 10.1093/neuonc/nou208.61

[68] Forsyth P, Roldán G, George D, Wallace C, Palmer CA, Morris D, et al. A phase I trial of intratumoral administration of reovirus in patients with histologically confirmed recurrent malignant gliomas. Molecular Therapy. 2008;**16**(3):627-632. DOI: 10.1038/sj.mt.6300403

Section 5

Manufacture

Chapter 5

Development, Engineering and Biological Characterization of Stirred Tank Bioreactors

Cedric Schirmer, Thomas Nussbaumer, Reto Schöb, Ralf Pörtner, Regine Eibl and Dieter Eibl

Additional information is available at the end of the chapter

http://dx.doi.org/10.5772/intechopen.79444

Abstract

Stirred tank bioreactors are still the predominant cultivation systems in large scale biopharmaceutical production. Today, several manufacturers provide both reusable and single-use systems, whereas the broad variety of designs and properties lead to deviations in biological performance. Although the methods for bioreactor characterization are well established, varying experimental conditions and procedures can result in significantly different outcomes. In order to guarantee a reliable comparison and evaluation of different single-use and reusable bioreactor types, standardized methods for their characterization are needed. Equally important is the biological capability of bioreactors, which must be accessed by standardized cultivation procedures of industrially relevant organisms (bacteria, yeasts as well as mammalian and animal cell cultures). In addition, the implementation of well-defined uniform procedures for biological and engineering characterization during the development phase can support a fast assessment of the suitability of a bioreactor system. Based on stirred bioreactors, we describe the aspects of the engineering characterization in order to discuss further the biological characterization as a valuable complement. Finally, a case study is presented.

Keywords: stirred bioreactor, characterization, mixing time, power input, volumetric mass transfer coefficient, development, cultivation system

1. Introduction

Stirred bioreactor systems have been used on a large scale since the beginning of antibiotics and insulin production, and are indispensable in biopharmaceutical production today [1]. They are the most frequently used bioreactor systems as they are suitable for various expression systems, currently using predominantly recombinant *Escherichia coli* (*E. coli*) strains or Chinese hamster ovary (CHO) cell lines [2–7].

Stirred bioreactors are available as reusable systems made of steel and glass or as single-use systems in different sizes. Many well-known manufacturers offer standard stainless steel systems with volumes from 2 to 1000 L, whereby larger systems with several cubic meters are also available according to customer specifications. The smaller scale glass bioreactors are used in research and process development [8]. The single-use systems, depending on their size, are either available as flexible bags or rigid vessels. They have become increasingly established in recent years and have found their way into biopharmaceutical productions with volumes of up to 2000 L. Eibl et al. [9] gives an overview of the currently available single-use systems.

In addition to the economic reasons for choosing one of the many reusable or single-use systems, they have to meet the requirements of the desired fermentation process. The design and equipment of stirred bioreactors differ in terms of their performance. The efficiency of the bioreactor is described with the help of process engineering parameters [10, 11]. Therefore, the mixing time θ_m of the system, the volumetric mass transfer coefficient k_La and the specific power input P/V are determined. This enables a comparison of different bioreactor types and the definition of suitable process parameters to achieve the desired product quality and quantity [12].

A new approach based on process engineering characterization is the biological characterization. This may be a standardized *E. coli* model process enabling a reveal in the performance limits of the bioreactor system.

It will be shown that process engineering characterization in combination with biological characterization is a simple standardized approach, which is not only necessary for the evaluation of existing bioreactor types, but also makes a valuable contribution during the development phase of new systems.

2. Theoretical background

The bioreactors used for the cultivation of microorganisms, mammalian and animal cells differ from reactors in the chemical industry in their aspect ratio (*H/D*). While *H/D* ratios of 1:1 occur in chemical production, these are usually 2:1 for bioreactors for cell cultures and 3:1 for microorganisms. The background to this is the longer residence time of oxygen or process air introduced into the system near the reactor bottom and the better temperature control due to the larger ratio of surface to volume [6, 10, 13]. However, with increasing reactor size, *H/D* ratios of up to 5:1 also occur [14]. For the cylindrical bioreactor vessel, the shape of the upper and lower end elements is also crucial. Curved heads with geometries from a hemisphere to a flat plate are used, whereby the dished head is the most common element. The reasons for this are the higher durability compared to planar end elements, and the geometry-related lower overall height compared to hemispherical elements. By avoiding dead zones and edges, cleaning of the system (hygienic design) and mixing is also favored. The upper end is usually a flat lid, which facilitates accessibility for the installation of probes or correction agents and feed [15, 16].

2.1. Agitation

Besides the vessel geometry, the impeller is the central element of the bioreactor. The choice of the right agitator organ has a decisive influence on the success of cultivation, as it prevents local sources and sinks. It is now possible to choose from a variety of different impeller designs, while taking into account the type of microorganism, human or animal cell line to be cultivated. Shear-sensitive cell culture processes are characterized by low energy and low oxygen input ($P/V \approx 5$–200 W·m^{-3}/$OTR \approx 0.5$–8 mmol O_2·L^{-1}·h^{-1}) as well as small cooling capacities. Axial flow impellers are often used for this purpose. For most applications with microorganisms, however, especially in the high cell density range (≈ 100 g·L^{-1} dry cell weight), higher specific power inputs and oxygen transfer rates are required ($P/V > 5$ kW·m^{-3} / $OTR \approx 300$–500 mmol O_2·L^{-1}·h^{-1}). For this purpose, radial flow impellers are used. Higher energy inputs lead to an improved gas dispersion and thus to higher oxygen transfer rates [6, 7, 10, 17–24]. Zlokarnik [19] and Mirro & Voll [17] provide an overview of the impeller types frequently used, and their field of application for the cultivation of various microbial and animal cell lines. Therefore, the process properties, in particular the mixing time, volumetric mass transfer coefficient and power input in combination with the resulting shear gradient are decisive for the impeller design to be selected [25]. Depending on the application and bioreactor size, multi-stage configurations with combinations of radial and axial flow impellers are also possible.

2.2. Drive

Traditionally, the agitator is driven via a centrally mounted shaft with the aid of a motor located above or below the bioreactor. The feedthrough of the shaft into the bioreactor has to be sealed. In the simplest case, a single-acting mechanical seal reduces the escape of organisms from the bioreactor, but bears the risk of contamination [16]. For reasons of product safety, as well as maintaining a tight containment, double mechanical seals are predominantly used. Two pairs of sliding rings are arranged one behind the other and form an intermediate space through which a barrier fluid flows. The pressurized barrier liquid, which is often sterile condensate, prevents leakage from the fermenter [26]. Magnetic couplings offer an alternative to complex double-acting mechanical seals. The magnetic field transfers the torque from the motor through the closed bioreactor to the impeller. The risk of contamination is further decreased by contactless power transmission [13]. In industrial applications, both free-floating and bearing-supported impellers can be found. Bearing-supported impellers are manufactured by MAVAG AG, Millipore Corporation and ZETA Holding GmbH, among others. The impeller with one part of the magnetic coupling sits on a bearing journal where the second part of the magnetic coupling is also located. The mounting is often done by means of ceramic plain bearings [27–29]. However, friction with insufficient lubrication may result in attrition of the material [30]. The levitation technology is used, for example, by Sartorius AG and Pall AG for mixing systems. Only the impeller with one part of the magnetic coupling is located in the vessel. The magnetic field applied causes the impeller to lift off the bottom of the container. This simple type of drive does not require a bearing, and is therefore ideally suited for use in single-use systems, whereas radially acting forces are difficult to absorb [31, 32]. As shown in our case study (see Section 3.1), the levitation technology is also suitable for new stirred bioreactors.

2.3. Characterization according to parametric and experimental approaches

Due to the large number of bioreactors available and their different process engineering properties, the choice of the right system for the requirements of a desired and successful process is decisive. The process engineering characterization allows the comparison of different systems and supports process optimization and scale-up strategies by using parametric as well as experimental approaches [11, 12]. Therefore in January 2016, DECHEMA issued a recommendation with standardized methods for obtaining reliable experimental data, which can be applied to both reusable and single-use bioreactor systems [33].

The dimensionless Reynolds number describes the ratio of inertial to viscous forces in a flow and describes it as laminar, transient or turbulent (Re_{crit} 1–10·10^4) [34, 35]. For stirred bioreactor systems, the Reynolds number can be determined parametrically as a function of the impeller speed N, the impeller diameter d, the density ρ and the viscosity η according to Eq. (1).

$$Re = \frac{\rho \cdot N \cdot d^2}{\eta} \tag{1}$$

Another parameter is the maximum fluid velocity (u_{max}), which usually corresponds to the tip speed u_{tip} (Eq. (2)).

$$u_{tip} = \pi \cdot d \cdot N \tag{2}$$

In order to avoid sources and sinks in the bioreactor, a homogeneous distribution of all components is required. A benchmark of homogeneity is the mixing quality, which is regarded as adequate at 95% [36]. The mixing time θ_m defines the time required after adding a disturbance variable to the system (e.g. change in temperature, concentration, conductivity or density) to achieve the required mixing quality [12, 35, 36]. Eq. (3) applies in completely turbulent flows, in which case the mixing number c_H is calculated according to Eq. (4).

$$\theta_m \propto (P/V)^{-1/3} \tag{3}$$

$$c_H = \theta_m \cdot N = \text{const.} \tag{4}$$

One of the most important parameters is the specific power input P/V, as this is responsible for maintaining sufficient mixing and mass transfer. There are several methods for determining the power input. The most common is the direct torque measurement [12, 37]. For the calculation according to Eq. (5), the effective impeller torque (difference between the torque when stirring in liquid M and the dead torque in air M_d) will be measured by means of a torque sensor. If a DC motor with a known motor torque constant K_t is used, it is also possible to determine the respective torque by measuring the required current I and using Eq. (6) [38].

$$P/V = \frac{(M - M_d) \cdot 2 \cdot \pi \cdot N}{V} \tag{5}$$

$$M = K_t \cdot I \tag{6}$$

Oxygen supply is essential for aerobic cultivation processes. This is ensured by the use of spargers, gassing via membranes or the fluid surface [21, 39]. The oxygen transition is defined by the oxygen transfer rate (*OTR*) and depends on the mixing efficiency, the power input, the gassing rate and the fluid properties [40, 41]. It results from the product of the mass transfer coefficient k_L and the volume-specific interface area a as well as the oxygen concentration difference $c^*_{O_2} - c_{O_2}$ as the driving force (Eq. (7)).

$$\frac{d\,C_{O_2}}{dt} = OTR = k_L a \cdot \left(C^*_{O_2} - C_{O_2}\right) \tag{7}$$

2.4. Characterization by biological approaches

Biological characterization focuses on the evaluation and comparison of bioreactor systems with respect to their biological performance. With the help of a model organism, it should be possible to make an exact prediction of the suitability of a bioreactor system for a desired purpose with a standardized cultivation procedure [42]. For example, two biological test procedures with respiratory yeast and mycelium-forming fungi were developed by Adler and Fiechter [43] and Wagner [44], since the physical characterization often only provides information about optimal bioreactor design conditions and information for improved scale transfer. For this reason, DECHEMA's *'Single-use technology in biopharmaceutical production'* working group is currently working on a new standardized procedure for the biological characterization of classical stirred bioreactors and single-use systems using batch and fed-batch cultivations in addition to the recommendation for process engineering characterization. *Escherichia coli* W3110 is used as a model organism. This is a subspecies of the *E. coli* K12 strain, which is one of the most frequently used and best characterized microorganisms. The suitability of *E. coli* as a model organism can be explained by its high availability, short generation time and extensively investigated growth behavior as well as its high relevance in the biopharmaceutical industry [20, 45, 46].

3. Case study

In this case study, the methodical procedures described above are used to develop a bearing-free magnetically driven 2 L benchtop bioreactor system, which is based on Levitronix's freely levitating impeller technology.

3.1. Bioreactor and setup

The use of a magnetic drive without bearings enables the establishment of a seal-free, contactless and magnetically mounted bottom impeller, which offers an almost unlimited speed range and a minimized risk of contamination (**Figure 1**).

The impeller levitating in the bioreactor at the bottom creates a constant gap, which is made possible by the passive stabilization of the stirring element by a constantly changing magnetic field [47, 48]. For design reasons, a flat end element was chosen for the bottom, into which the BPS-i30 and BPS-i100 drives from Levitronix GmbH were introduced for the investigations. A glass cylinder with a diameter of 124.5 mm and a planar lid with nozzles for probes and the

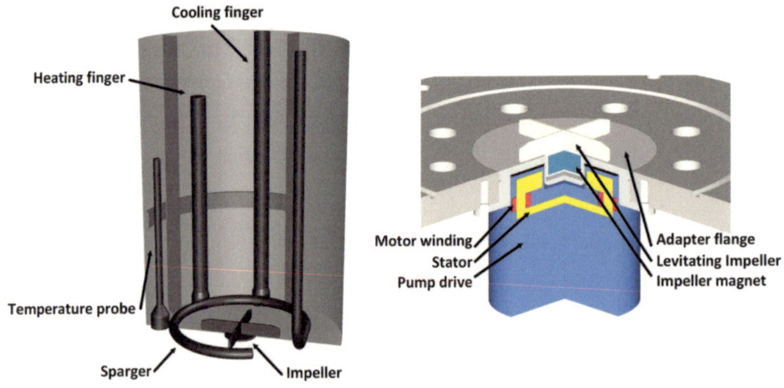

Figure 1. Setup and design of 2 L vessel (left) and construction of the designed impeller unit in the bioreactor bottom plate (right).

possibility of adding correction agents and feed solutions was mounted on top of it. The impellers used for the BPS-i30 drive are the geometries shown in **Figure 2** with diameters of 20, 30, 40 and 50 mm and, based on this, 40, 50, 60 and 74 mm for the more powerful BPS-i100 drive. The oxygen input was made possible by means of a ring sparger with holes facing upwards. The temperature was controlled by using an electric heating and a water-flow cooling finger.

3.2. Process engineering characterization

All process engineering parameters to be investigated were determined by means of design of experiments, and the experimental data were evaluated using MODDE 10.1 (Umetrics, Sweden).

3.2.1. Power input

The specific power input (non-gassed conditions) was determined with water at a constant temperature of 25°C, and a maximum working volume according to Ref. [33]. Because of the constructive conditions of the vessel and motor geometry, the sensor method for determining the torque was not applicable. Due to the known motor constants K_t with 1.13 and 2.0 Ncm·A^{-1} (BPS-i30/BPS-i100), the torque can be recalculated with the desired current for agitation using Eqs. (5) and (6). Likewise, the examined torque of the empty vessel (dead weight torque) was subtracted from the measured torque of the filled vessel.

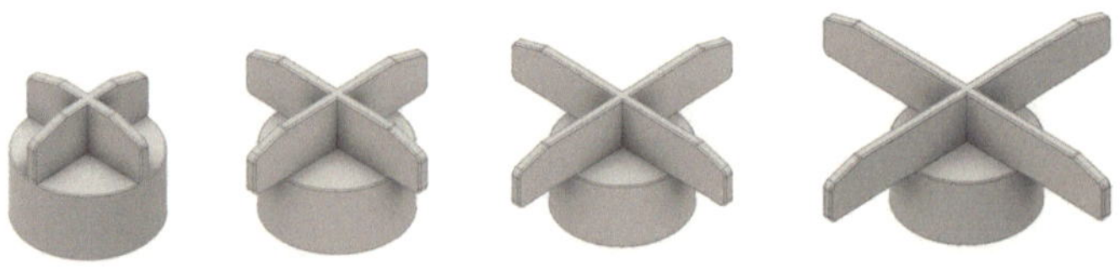

Figure 2. Magnetic impeller with increasing blade diameter.

Additionally, the torque was determined by numerical simulations (computational fluid dynamics (CFD)). Based on the predicted fluid flow, the power inputs of the impellers were obtained from the torque acting on the impeller and the shaft. Therefore, the fluid flow inside the bioreactor equipped with the different impellers was modeled using the finite volume solver ANSYS Fluent (ANSYS Inc., Version 16.2, USA) by using the realizable k-ϵ turbulence model for water at 25°C [49]. The vessel walls and the impeller were treated as non-slip boundaries with standard wall functions. The axial velocity at the fluid surface was set to zero. All equations were discretized using the first-order upwind scheme and the COUPLED algorithm was chosen for pressure-velocity coupling. The fluid domain was discretized by an unstructured mesh consisting of about 8×10^6 to 11×10^6 tetrahedrons.

3.2.2. *Mixing time*

The mixing times were examined by the decolorization method (iodometry) at maximum working volume according to [33]. Therefore, the bioreactor was filled with water and 2 mL·L^{-1} iodine potassium iodide solution (potassium iodide 40 g·L^{-1}, iodine 20 g·L^{-1}) and 5 mL·L^{-1} starch solution (1% w/v) were added under agitation at a constant temperature of 25°C. After ensuring a completely homogeneous chemical solution and a quasi-stationary fluid flow pattern, 4 mL·L^{-1} sodium thiosulfate solution were added and the time was measured until the color change from dark blue to colorless was achieved.

3.2.3. *Volumetric mass transfer coefficient*

The $k_L a$ values were determined by the gassing-out method with phosphate-buffered saline (PBS) at 37°C for gassing rates between 0.5 and 2 vvm with a maximum working volume according to Ref. [33]. An OIM-PSt3 probe in combination with a prototype sensor (OEC-PSt3-UF) without protection membrane (PreSens GmbH, Germany, sensor response time 4 s) was used for measurement of dissolved oxygen *DO*. For a measurement, a quasi-stationary fluid flow pattern was ensured and the dissolved oxygen in the PBS in the bioreactor was eliminated by introducing nitrogen. Afterwards, the data acquisition was started, the nitrogen supply stopped, the process air supply set to the desired aeration rate and the aeration started. The measurement was completed when a saturated oxygen concentration had been reached, indicated by a stable *DO* value of 100%. The evaluation and calculation of the $k_L a$ value according to Meusel et al. [33] was done for a *DO* saturation rate between 10 and 90%.

3.3. Biological characterization

Based on the results of the process engineering characterization, the process parameters for the *E. coli* cultivations were set to values resulting in the highest $k_L a$ values by maintaining a constant gassing and tip speed of 2 vvm (process air) and 7000 and 2900 rpm (20 mm – BPS-i30/40 mm – BPS-i100). Therefore, a cryopreserved culture of *E. coli* W3110 thyA36 supO λ- (ATCC: 27325) was incubated for 24 h at 37°C on lysogenic broth (LB) agar. Pre-culture 1 (1-L baffled shake flask, Corning, USA) was inoculated in 200 mL LB medium with one colony from the petri dish and incubated for 8 h at 37°C in a shaking incubator.

The second pre-culture was also incubated in a 1-L shake flask with 150 mL medium at an initial optical density at 600 nm (*OD600*) of 0.1 for 16 h at 30°C in a shaker. The medium of the second pre- and main culture correspond to the composition described by Biener et al. [50] with concentrations ($g{\cdot}L^{-1}$): glucose (pre-culture 2: 10, batch: 80 and fed-batch: 20), $MgSO_4{\cdot}7H_2O$ (0.54), $(NH_4)_2H$-citrat (1.01), Na_2SO_4 (2.02), $(NH_4)_2SO_4$ (4.03), NH_4Cl (0.51), K_2HPO_4 (15.17), $NaH_2PO_4{\cdot}H_2O$ (3.55), $CaCl_2{\cdot}2H_2O$ (2.25 10^{-3}), $ZnSO_4{\cdot}7H_2O$ ($0.81{\cdot}10^{-3}$), $MnSO_4{\cdot}H_2O$ ($0.45{\cdot}10^{-3}$), Na_2-EDTA$\cdot 2H_2O$ ($45{\cdot}10^{-3}$), $FeCl_3{\cdot}6H_2O$ ($37.6{\cdot}10^{-3}$), $CuSO_4{\cdot}5H_2O$ ($0.72{\cdot}10^{-3}$) and $CoCl_2{\cdot}6H_2O$ ($0.81{\cdot}10^{-3}$).

For the fed-batch process, a concentrated feed with a high glucose concentration was added into the bioreactor after the initial glucose had depleted. To maintain a constant growth rate, an exponential profile was used [51, 52]. The feed medium was formulated with the following concentrations ($g{\cdot}L^{-1}$): glucose (655.3), $MgSO_4{\cdot}7H_2O$ (16.02), $CaCl_2{\cdot}2H_2O$ ($43{\cdot}10^{-3}$), $ZnSO_4{\cdot}7H_2O$ ($15{\cdot}10^{-3}$), $MnSO_4{\cdot}H_2O$ ($85{\cdot}10^{-3}$), Na_2-EDTA$\cdot 2H_2O$ ($85{\cdot}10^{-3}$), $FeCl_3{\cdot}6H_2O$ ($71{\cdot}10^{-3}$), $CuSO_4{\cdot}5H_2O$ ($14{\cdot}10^{-3}$) and $CoCl_2{\cdot}6H_2O$ ($15{\cdot}10^{-3}$). In contrast to the batch process, the *DO* was regulated by the substitution of process air with pure oxygen.

The batch fermentations had a starting volume of 2 L, whereas the fed-batch started with 1.3 L to ensure an appropriate covering of all sensors and heating and cooling devices. After reaching an *OD600* of 150, a second feed with $(NH_4)_2HPO_4$ was immediately added to a concentration of 4 $g{\cdot}L^{-1}$ to the bioreactor. The pH was regulated automatically by adding 20% (w/w) ammonia solution and foaming was controlled by the addition of 1:5 diluted Antifoam 204 (Sigma-Aldrich). Cultivations were terminated at $DO \approx 0\%$.

3.4. Results

In the run-up to the experimental investigations, the new bioreactor system with the magnetic drive was numerically examined with regard to the process engineering parameters regarding its suitability for the cultivation of microorganisms. As expected, the specific power input shows an exponential increase with rising rotational speed (**Figure 3**). However, it also becomes apparent that with the weaker BPS-i30 drive, only the impellers with a diameter of 20 and 30 mm are in the range of microbial requirements with $P/V > 5$ $kW{\cdot}m^{-3}$ and $u_{tip} > 1.5$ $m{\cdot}s^{-1}$ [10]. With the more powerful BPS-i100 drive, this is the case for all impellers.

The experimentally determined specific power inputs show only minor deviations compared to the numerically determined values, whereby larger differences result in increasing rotational speed. The largest deviation for the 20 mm impeller at 7000 rpm ($u_{tip} = 7.3$ $m{\cdot}s^{-1}$) is around 3.5 $kW{\cdot}m^{-3}$. This circumstance can result from the radial forces not taken into account in the simulations, which increase with rising rotational speed due to possible impeller imbalances. Therefore, in the present case, the power inputs are estimated as slightly too low with the help of the CFD.

With regard to the mixing time, **Figure 4** shows that all impellers with a specific power input of 1 $kW{\cdot}m^{-3}$ and above meet a required mixing time of $\theta_m < 10$ s [53]. A turbulent flow regime with $Re > Re_{crit}$ is also present from this value on (see **Table 1**). The slope of the regressions of the mixing times is between −0.19 and − 0.4, which is close to the theoretical value of −0.33 (see Eq. (3)). Thus, mixing numbers in the range of 65–183 result according to Eq. (4).

http://dx.doi.org/10.5772/intechopen.79444

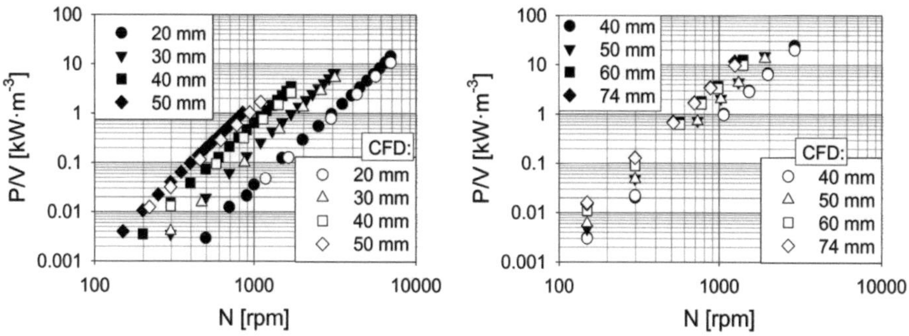

Figure 3. Double logarithmic representation of the numerically and experimentally determined P/V values for all used impellers as a function of N (left: BPS-i30/right: BPS-i100). P/V, specific power input; N, impeller speed.

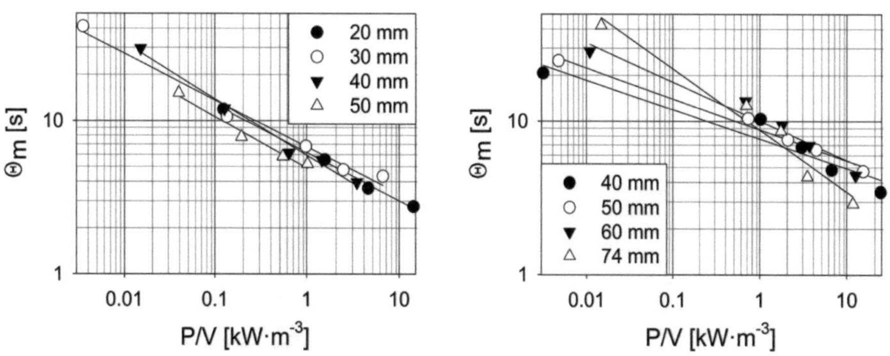

Figure 4. Double logarithmic representation of the experimentally determined θ_m values for all impellers used as a function of P/V (left: BPS-i30/right: BPS-i100). θ_m, mixing time; P/V, specific power input.

The experimentally determined k_La values for the two impellers 20 and 40 mm (BPS-i30/BPS-i100) are shown in **Figure 5**. The values explain the highest volumetric mass transfer coefficients found at the highest possible rotational speeds of 7000 and 2900 rpm (14.3 kW·m^{-3}/24.4 kW·m^{-3}) (see **Table 1**). The strong influence of the impeller speed becomes clear, as at low rotational speeds most of the gas reaches the fluid surface with very low dispersion due to the insurmountable buoyancy force of the introduced gas. This effect is often also referred to as "flooding" [35, 54], whereby in the present bioreactor design, the impeller running on the bottom does not pull down the bubbles emerged by the higher lying sparger, and is therefore not able to disperse them sufficiently due to radially acting forces. Compared with experiments on the 30 and 100 L scale, the value determined with the 20 mm impeller is three times smaller [42].

Based on the process engineering investigations, the cultivation for biological characterization was carried out. The impellers 20 and 40 mm (BPS-i30/BPS-i100) used demonstrated identical behavior during the process up to hour 6 with respect to biomass, glucose and acetate concentrations as well as in the *DO* profile (see **Figure 6**). This can also be seen in the growth rates, which after approximately 3 h reach a value of $\mu \approx 0.4\ h^{-1}$. Due to the high glucose concentration, which inhibits growth with values of more than 50 g·L^{-1} [24], the maximum growth rate

Impeller diameter [mm]	BPS-i30		BPS-i100		*Re* at *P*/*V* of 1 W·m^{-3}
	N_{max} [rpm]	k_La [h^{-1}]	N_{max} [rpm]	k_La [h^{-1}]	
20	7000	206	—	—	≈ 19,900
30	3150	142	—	—	≈ 25,400
40	1700	172	2900	694	≈ 30,000
50	1100	170	1900	657	≈ 34,000
60	—	—	1400	560	≈ 37,000
74	—	—	1250	591	≈ 52,200

k_La, volumetric mass transfer coefficient; N_{max}, maximum impeller speed; Re, Reynolds number; P/V, specific power input.

Table 1. Representation of the highest experimentally determined k_La values (n = 5) for both drive systems used with the corresponding maximum impeller speeds and Reynolds numbers of the different impellers at a P/V of 1 W·m^{-3}.

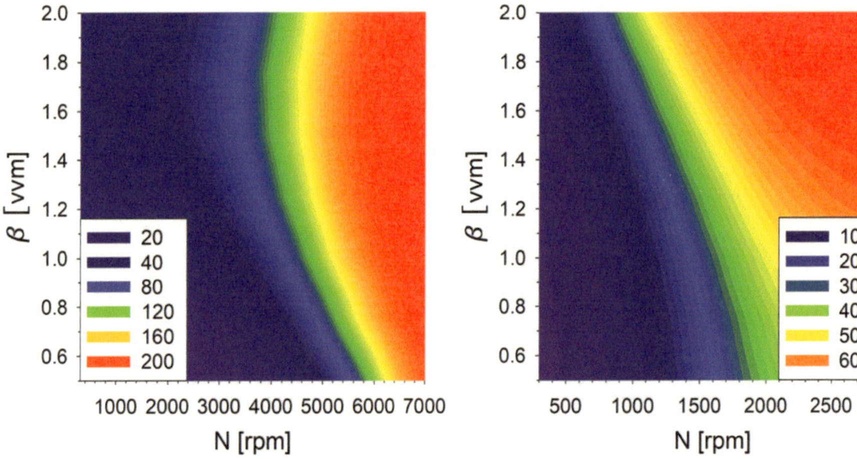

Figure 5. Representation of the experimentally determined k_La values (n = 5) as a function of N and β (left: BPS-i30, 20 mm, R^2 = 0.76/right: BPS-i100, 40 mm, R^2 = 0.96). k_La, volumetric mass transfer coefficient; N, impeller speed; β, gassing rate.

of 0.61 h^{-1} for this *E. coli* strain is not reached [45]. From hour 6, the use of the smaller impeller shows a successive decrease in the growth rate and a faster increase in acetate. This effect is ascribed to the lower oxygen content in the medium and a so-called salt effect by the increased addition of base, which could be observed during fermentation [24, 55–57]. This finally leads to a decrease in growth and glucose consumption, as acetate concentrations from 2 g·L^{-1} can have an inhibiting effect [58]. Thus, when using the smaller impeller, an *OD600* of 35.4 ± 0.1 or a dry cell weight DCW of 13.0 ± 1.8 g·L^{-1} is achieved. When using the larger impeller in combination with a more powerful drive and a resulting higher k_La value, an optical density of 65.3 ± 3.4 (21.6 ± 1.9 g·L^{-1} *DCW*) is reached.

http://dx.doi.org/10.5772/intechopen.79444

In reusable pilot bioreactors for microbial applications with 30 and 100 L previously tested, only optical densities of 39 ± 5 at higher oxygen transport rates of 735 and 745 h^{-1} were obtained [42]. This fact can only be attributed to the considerably shorter mixing times of 2.77 and 3.47 s (20 mm/40 mm) in the 2 L scale shown here. These were determined in the mentioned larger systems with 8–10 s. The additional oxygen uptake rate *OUR* determined during cultivation with the 40 mm impeller shows a maximum of 256 $mmol·L^{-1}·h^{-1}$ (see **Figure 6**).

The results of the fed-batch cultivations with the BPS-i100 system presented in **Figure 7** show an expected higher biomass concentration with an *OD600* of 262.4 ± 0.3, which corresponds to a *DCW* of 86.6 ± 1.9 $g·L^{-1}$. Due to the lower glucose concentration in the starting medium, a growth rate of >0.6 h^{-1} could be achieved after 3 h. With a further steady decrease in glucose concentration, the growth rate drops to values between 0.3 and 0.4 h^{-1}, which were controlled by exponential feed addition. The feed was started between hours 6 and 7 since the glucose in the medium was depleted at this time, which is also expressed by the corresponding *DO* peak. To keep the oxygen content constant at 40% during the further cultivation, the process air was gradually substituted with oxygen from hour 7 on. From hour 12.5 on, 2 vvm pure oxygen was required. Interestingly, after a cultivation time of 11.5 h, there were signs of insufficient cooling of the system, as the bioreactor temperature rose steadily to a maximum of 40.7°C by the end of the cultivation.

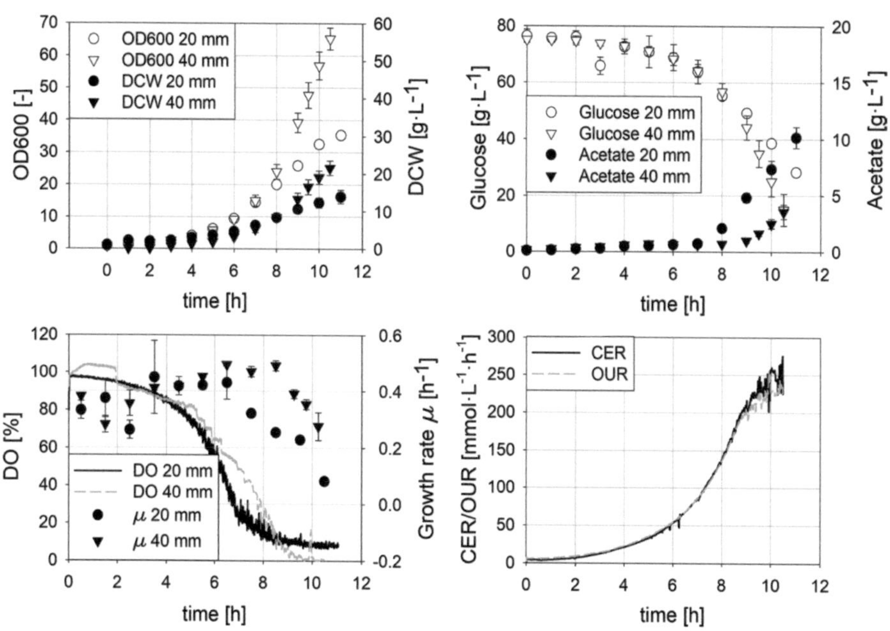

Figure 6. Determined biomass profiles for OD600 and DCW (top left), glucose and acetate concentrations (top right) and DO profiles as well as the growth rates (bottom left) over the process time from the batch cultures (n = 2) when using impellers with a diameter of 20 and 40 mm (BPS-i30/BPS-i100). The lower right diagram shows the OUR and CER determined in the exhaust air over the cultivation time for the latter bioreactor configuration (40 mm). OD600, optical density; DCW, dry cell weight; DO, dissolved oxygen; μ, growth rate; OUR, oxygen uptake rate; CER, carbon dioxide formation rate.

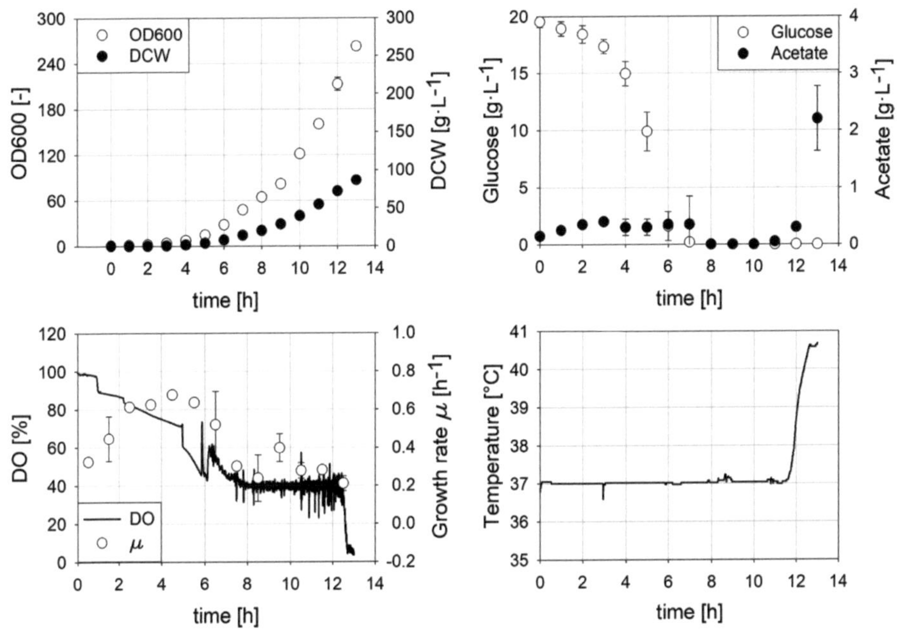

Figure 7. Certain biomass profiles for OD600 and DCW (top left), glucose and acetate concentrations (top right) and DO profile as well as the growth rates (bottom left) over the process time from the fed-batch cultures (n = 2) using the impeller with a diameter of and 40 mm (BPS-i100). The lower right diagram shows the temperature curve in the bioreactor over the cultivation time. OD600, optical density; DCW, dry cell weight; DO, dissolved oxygen; μ, growth rate.

4. Discussion

The determined process engineering parameters demonstrate that the newly developed bioreactor system can be used for the cultivation of shear-sensitive animal cells as well as microbial cells up to the high cell density range. In this way, the process engineering parameters for all impellers with specific power inputs of up to 500 W·m^{-3} show suitability for animal cell culture processes. The k_La values are within a range of 20 and 100 h^{-1}, and the resulting mixing times are ≤10 s. These are also typical values described in the literature for animal cell culture bioreactors, such as the Finesse SmartGlass bioreactor [59], the Mobius CellReady 3 L bioreactor [60] or the reusable BIOSTAT UniVessel and BIOSTAT UniVessel SU [11]. A first proof of concept batch cultivation with CHO XM 111-10 suspension cells (SEAP secreting cell line, the secreted alkaline phosphatase of the placenta, CCOS No. 837) in a chemically defined minimal medium using the BPS-i30 drive resulted in middle cell densities of up to $4{\cdot}10^6$ cells·mL^{-1}(data not shown), which are in the same order of magnitude as in the previously mentioned bioreactors, and in the BioBlu 0.3c as well as BIOSTAT® A [61–66]. Taking into account the shear stress acting on the cells, theoretically higher cell densities may also be achievable, since the performance limits of the system have not been reached, and can be complemented by suitable feeding strategies.

In addition, due to the simple design of the system, with the elimination of seals and bearings, by using a magnetic drive with a freely levitating impeller the bioreactor is almost maintenance-free and the risk of contamination is reduced. It also facilitates cleaning and the easy and fast change of impeller types for different applications. Furthermore, the bioreactor system offers a high turn down ratio allowing an easy-to-scale process.

While conventional microbial processes can also be implemented with the less powerful BPS-i30 drive, the BPS-i100 in combination with the 40 mm impeller is recommended for high cell density microbial processes. This is demonstrated by nearly a doubling of the optical densities in the *E. coli* batch cultivations, and the results of the fed-batch procedure.

So it comes as no surprise that the specific power inputs obtained in the case study with the new bioreactor provide comparable results to other microbial bioreactor systems described in the literature. For bioreactors with sizes of 1–100 L, these are between 2.5 and 20 $kW{\cdot}m^{-3}$ [42, 67–69], whereby a minimum requirement of >5 $kW{\cdot}m^{-3}$ is generally assumed [10]. The achieved mixing numbers are partly $c_H > 100$ due to the impeller position at the vessel bottom, which are above the usual values for bioreactors equipped with different impeller types [35]. Mixing times are also below the 10 s recommended for microbial requirements [53], as is also the case in other conventional bioreactors up to pilot scale [42, 70, 71]. However, compared to systems with larger volumes, a possible increase in mixing time of up to 2 min must also be taken into account [10]. According to manufacturers and previously published data, for several bioreactors k_La values between 300 and 745 h^{-1} are reached and are sufficient for microbial processes with a resulting *OTR* from 250 to 500 $mmol{\cdot}L^{-1}{\cdot}h^{-1}$ [20, 42, 67, 69, 70, 72–74]. Against this background, only the impellers with the BPS-i100 drive shown in the case study appear to be relevant for microbial industrial processes. The impellers driven on the bioreactor bottom with the weaker BPS-i30 drive are not able to disperse the gas bubbles sufficiently. In conventional bioreactors, this problem is circumvented by the fact that the impellers are located above the aeration organ. So far, the fed-batch cultures have shown, one of the main problems of microbial high cell density cultures is the removal of the heat generated in the system, which means that this either has to be countered with larger heat exchange surfaces or lower coolant temperatures [10]. Nevertheless, with the performed fed-batch model process, a higher cell density (>260) could be achieved as in other microbial systems. These given results of *OD600* values between 100 and 201 in a very similar high-demanding *E. coli* process [67, 70, 72, 74, 75].

5. Conclusion

The combination of DECHEMA's recommendation for process engineering characterization and the *E. coli* standard model process described above provides an easy-to-implement approach for the standardized qualification of existing microbial bioreactor systems, and for those currently under development, as shown for the novel benchtop-scale bioreactor equipped with Levitronix's magnetic drives.

The investigated process engineering parameters allow the estimation of its optimal working areas and limits. In addition, it allows a selection of a suitable impeller design to increase the productivity of biopharmaceutical processes. The impeller with a diameter of 40 mm in combination with the more powerful BPS-i100 drive shows the highest k_La value and a mixing time of <4 s at the highest specific power input of 24.4 $kW{\cdot}m^{-3}$. In line with expectations, the largest biomass with an optical density of 65.3 in batch mode and 262.4 in fed-batch mode is achieved.

Surprisingly, the use of the smallest impeller with the smaller BPS-i30 drive shows a comparable biomass concentration to bioreactors on a pilot scale despite a very low k_La value for microbial processes. This circumstance is not foreseeable by the sole process engineering characterization, so that the additional use of a biological characterization approach becomes evident. The suitability of the presented developed bioreactor concept for microbial applications could be clearly demonstrated, even if it seems rather unusual in comparison to commercial systems due to its bottom drive without bearings. The complete characterization provides the possibility for an easier transfer to the industrial biopharmaceutical scale. Finally, the currently available bioengineering data of the new developed bioreactor indicate that the bioreactor operated with the BPS-i30 drive can also be used to grow animal cells. More detailed investigations are planned in the future.

Abbreviations

CCOS	culture collection of Switzerland
CFD	computational fluid dynamics
CHO	Chinese hamster ovary cell line
CHO XM 111–10	SEAP secreting cell line
E. coli	*Escherichia coli*
LB	lysogenic broth
PBS	phosphate-buffered saline
SEAP	secreted alkaline phosphatase of the placenta

Nomenclature

c_{O_2}	present oxygen concentration [mmol·L^{-1}]
$c^*_{O_2}$	maximum oxygen concentration [mmol·L^{-1}]
μ	specific growth rate [h^{-1}]
a	phase boundary interface [m^{-1}]
c_H	mixing number [–]
d	impeller diameter [m]
D	vessel diameter [m]
DCW	dry cell weight [g·L^{-1}]
DO	dissolved oxygen [%]
H	vessel height [m]

H/D	ratio of vessel height to diameter [–]
I	current [A]
k_L	mass transfer coefficient [m·h^{-1}]
k_La	volumetric mass transfer coefficient [h^{-1}]
K_t	motor torque constant [N·m·A^{-1}]
M	torque [N·m]
M_d	dead weight torque [N·m]
N	number of impeller revolutions [rps]
$OD600$	optical density at 600 nm [–]
OTR	oxygen transfer rate [mmol·L^{-1}·h^{-1}]
OUR	oxygen uptake rate [mmol·L^{-1}·h^{-1}]
P/V	specific power input [W·m^{-3}]
R^2	regression coefficient [–]
Re	Reynolds number [–]
u_{tip}	tip speed [m·s^{-1}]
V	volume [L]
β	gassing rate [vvm]
η	viscosity [Pa·s]
θ_m	mixing time [s]
π	3.14159 [–]
ρ	density [kg·m^{-3}]

Author details

Cedric Schirmer[1]*, Thomas Nussbaumer[2], Reto Schöb[2], Ralf Pörtner[3], Regine Eibl[1] and Dieter Eibl[1]

*Address all correspondence to: cedric.schirmer@zhaw.ch

1 School of Life Sciences and Facility Management, Institute of Chemistry and Biotechnology, Zurich University of Applied Sciences, Wädenswil, Switzerland

2 Levitronix GmbH, Zurich, Switzerland

3 Institute of Bioprocess and Biosystems Engineering, Hamburg University of Technology, Hamburg, Germany

References

[1] Meyer H-P, Schmidhalter DR. The history and economic relevance of industrial scale suspension culture of living cells. In: Meyer H-P, Schmidhalter DR, editors. Industrial Scale Suspension Culture of Living Cells. Weinheim, Germany: Wiley-VCH Verlag GmbH & Co. KGaA; 2014. pp. 1-38. DOI: 10.1002/9783527683321.ch00

[2] Schmidt FR. Recombinant expression systems in the pharmaceutical industry. Applied Microbiology and Biotechnology. 2004;**65**(4):363-372. DOI: 10.1007/s00253-004-1656-9

[3] Terpe K. Overview of bacterial expression systems for heterologous protein production: From molecular and biochemical fundamentals to commercial systems. Applied Microbiology and Biotechnology. 2006;**72**(2):211-222. DOI: 10.1007/s00253-006-0465-8

[4] Butler M. Animal cell cultures: Recent achievements and perspectives in the production of biopharmaceuticals. Applied Microbiology and Biotechnology. 2005;**68**(3):283-291. DOI: 10.1007/s00253-005-1980-8

[5] Butler M, Meneses-Acosta A. Recent advances in technology supporting biopharmaceutical production from mammalian cells. Applied Microbiology and Biotechnology. 2012;**96**(4):885-894. DOI: 10.1007/s00253-012-4451-z

[6] Chmiel H. Bioreaktoren. In: Bioprozesstechnik. Heidelberg: Spektrum Akademischer Verlag; 2011. pp. 197-236. DOI: 10.1007/978-3-8274-2477-8_7

[7] Pörtner R. Bioreactors for mammalian cells. In: Al-Rubeai M, editor. Animal Cell Culture. Cham: Springer; 2015. pp. 89-135. DOI: 10.1007/978-3-319-10320-4_4

[8] Clapp KP, Castan A, Lindskog EK. Upstream processing equipment. In: Jagschies G, Lindskog E, Lacki K, Galliher PM, editors. Biopharmaceutical Processing. Oxford: Elsevier; 2018. pp. 457-476. DOI: 10.1016/B978-0-08-100623-8.00024-4

[9] Eibl R, Jossen V, Eibl D. Einweg-Bioreaktoren. Chemie unserer Zeit. 2018:2-9. DOI: 10.1002/ciuz.201800803

[10] Jossen V, Eibl R, Pörtner R, Kraume M, Eibl D. Stirred bioreactors. In: Larroche C, Angeles Sanroman M, Du G, Ashok P, editors. Current Developments in Biotechnology and Bioengineering. Amsterdam: Elsevier; 2017. pp. 179-215. DOI: 10.1016/B978-0-444-63663-8.00007-0

[11] Löffelholz C, Kaiser SC, Kraume M, Eibl R, Eibl D. Dynamic single-use bioreactors used in modern liter- and m^3-scale biotechnological processes: Engineering characteristics and scaling up. In: Eibl D, Eibl R, editors. Disposable Bioreactors II. Berlin, Heidelberg: Springer Berlin Heidelberg; 2013. pp. 1-44. DOI: 10.1007/10_2013_187

[12] Löffelholz C, Husemann U, Greller G, Meusel W, Kauling J, Ay P, et al. Bioengineering parameters for single-use bioreactors: Overview and evaluation of suitable methods. Chemie Ingenieur Technik. 2013 Feb;**85**(1-2):40-56. DOI: 10.1002/cite.201200125

[13] Menkel F, editor. Einführung in die Technik von Bioreaktoren. München: Oldenbourg Wissenschaftsverlag; 1992. p. 234

[14] Chisti Y. Bioreactor design. In: Ratledge C, Kristiansen B, editors. Basic Biotechnology. Cambridge: Cambridge University Press; 2006. pp. 181-200. DOI: 10.1017/CBO9780-511802409.009

[15] Gleich D, Weyl R. Abschlusselemente. In: Apparateelemente. Berlin/Heidelberg: Springer-Verlag; 2006. p. 117-190. (VDI-Buch). DOI: 10.1007/3-540-30376-6_6

[16] Hinrichs J, Buck H, Hauser G. Sterilisation und Sterildesign. In: Chmiel H, editor. Bioprozesstechnik. Heidelberg: Spektrum Akademischer Verlag; 2011. pp. 237-262. DOI: 10.1007/978-3-8274-2477-8_8

[17] Mirro R, Voll K. Which impeller is right for your cell line? Bioprocess International. 2009;**7**(1):52-57

[18] Krahe M. Biochemical engineering. In: Ullmann's Encyclopedia of Industrial Chemistry. Weinheim, Germany: Wiley-VCH Verlag GmbH & Co. KGaA; 2003. pp. 549-618. DOI: 10.1002/14356007.b04_381

[19] Zlokarnik M. Stirring, general. In: Stirring. Weinheim, Germany: Wiley-VCH Verlag GmbH; 2001. pp. 1-75. DOI: 10.1002/9783527612703.ch01

[20] Sagmeister P, Jazini M, Klein J, Herwig C. Bacterial suspension cultures. In: Meyer H, Schmidhalter DR, editors. Industrial Scale Suspension Culture of Living Cells. Weinheim, Germany: Wiley-VCH Verlag GmbH & Co. KGaA; 2014. pp. 40-93. DOI: 10.1002/9783527683321.ch01

[21] Xing Z, Kenty BM, Li ZJ, Lee SS. Scale-up analysis for a CHO cell culture process in large-scale bioreactors. Biotechnology and Bioengineering. 2009 Jul 1;**103**(4):733-746. DOI: 10.1002/bit.22287

[22] Platas Barradas O, Jandt U, Da Minh PL, Villanueva M, Rath A, Reichl U, et al. Criteria for bioreactor comparison and operation standardisation during process development for mammalian cell culture. BMC Proceedings. 2011;**5**(Suppl 8):P47. DOI: 10.1186/1753-6561-5-S8-P47

[23] Ozturk SS. Engineering challenges in high density cell culture systems. Cytotechnology. 1996;**22**(1-3):3-16. DOI: 10.1007/BF00353919

[24] Riesenberg D. High-cell-density cultivation of *Escherichia coli*. Current Opinion in Biotechnology. 1991 Jun;**2**(3):380-384. DOI: 10.1016/S0958-1669(05)80142-9

[25] Xia J-Y, Wang Y-H, Zhang S-L, Chen N, Yin P, Zhuang Y-P, et al. Fluid dynamics investigation of variant impeller combinations by simulation and fermentation experiment. Biochemical Engineering Journal. 2009 Mar;**43**(3):252-260. DOI: 10.1016/j.bej.2008.10.010

[26] Wegel S, Heine H. Maßnahmen für den sicheren Umgang mit biologischen Agenzien im Produktionsbereich. In: Adelmann S, Schulze-Halberg H, editors. Arbeitsschutz in

Biotechnologie und Gentechnik. Berlin, Heidelberg: Springer Berlin Heidelberg; 1996. pp. 385-444. DOI: 10.1007/978-3-642-60942-8_7

[27] Mavag AG. MAVADRIVE® [Internet]. Available from: http://mavag.com.gutenberg.ch-meta.net/_wys_files/MAVADRIVE Broschuere.pdf [Accessed: 2018 May 15]

[28] ZETA Biopharma. ZETA magnetic agitators [Internet]. Available from: https://www.zeta.com/en/0uploads/dateienEnglisch450.pdf [Accessed: 2018 May 15]

[29] Millipore Corporation. NovAseptic Mixers [Internet]. Available from: http://www.sterileprocesscomponents.com/brochures/PB1200EN00_Mixers.pdf [Accessed: 2018 May 15]

[30] Haberhauer H, Bodenstein F. Elemente der drehenden Bewegung. In: Maschinenelemente. Berlin, Heidelberg: Springer Berlin Heidelberg; 2014. pp. 283-433. DOI: 10.1007/978-3-642-37417-3_4

[31] Pall Corporation. LevMixer® System [Internet]. 2018. Available from: https://shop.pall.com/INTERSHOP/web/WFS/PALL-PALLUS-Site/en_US/-/USD/ViewProductAttachment-OpenFile?LocaleId=&DirectoryPath=pdfs%2FBiopharmaceuticals&FileName=16-6543_USD2952b_LevMixer_SS.pdf&UnitName=PALL [Accessed: 2018 Mar 20]

[32] Sartorius Stedim Biotech GmbH. Brochure Standard Flexel® for LevMixer® 50 L to 1,000 L [Internet]. Available from: http://www.wisterchina.com/images/nr/201409/0710/3919421r5le1243xa3.pdf [Accessed: 2018 May 15]

[33] Meusel W, Löffelholz C, Husemann U, Dreher T, Greller G, Kauling J, et al. Recommendations for Process Engineering Characterisation of Single-Use Bioreactors and Mixing Systems by using Experimental Methods. Frankfurt am Main: DECHEMA; 2016. p. 31

[34] Nienow AW. Scale-up, stirred tank reactors. In: Flickinger MC, editor. Encyclopedia of Industrial Biotechnology. Hoboken, NJ, USA: John Wiley & Sons, Inc.; 2010. pp. 1-14. DOI: 10.1002/9780470054581.eib535

[35] Liepe F, Sperling R, Jembere S. Rührwerke: Theoretische Grundlagen, Auslegung und Bewertung. Köthen: Eigenverlag Fachhochschule; 1998. 548 p

[36] Kraume M. Mischen und Rühren. Weinheim, FRG: Wiley-VCH Verlag GmbH & Co. KGaA; 2002. 444 p. DOI: 10.1002/3527603360

[37] Ascanio G, Castro B, Galindo E. Measurement of power consumption in stirred vessels—A review. Chemical Engineering Research and Design. 2004;**82**(9):1282-1290. DOI: 10.1205/cerd.82.9.1282.44164

[38] Electro-Craft Corporation. DC Motors, Speed Controls, Servo Systems: An Engineering Handbook. Elsevier; 1972. 504 p

[39] Noack U, De Wilde D, Verhoeye F, Balbirnie E, Kahlert W, Adams T, et al. Single-use stirred tank reactor BIOSTAT CultiBag STR: Characterization and applications. In: Eibl R, Eibl D, editors. Single-Use Technology in Biopharmaceutical Manufacture. Hoboken, NJ, USA: John Wiley & Sons, Inc.; 2011. pp. 225-240. DOI: 10.1002/9780470909997.ch19

[40] Garcia-Ochoa F, Gomez E. Bioreactor scale-up and oxygen transfer rate in microbial processes: An overview. Biotechnology Advances. 2009;**27**(2):153-176. DOI: 10.1016/j.biotechadv.2008.10.006

[41] Van't Riet K. Review of measuring methods and results in nonviscous gas-liquid mass transfer in stirred vessels. Industrial and Engineering Chemistry Process Design and Development. 1979 Jul;**18**(3):357-364. DOI: 10.1021/i260071a001

[42] Schirmer C, Blaschczok K, Husemann U, Leupold M, Zahnow C, Rupprecht J, et al. Standardized qualification of stirred bioreactors for microbial biopharmaceutical production processes. Chemie Ingenieur Technik. 2017 Dec;**89**(12):1766-1772. DOI: 10.1002/cite.201700039

[43] Adler I, Fiechter A. Charakterisierung von Bioreaktoren mit biologischen Testsystemen. Chemie Ingenieur Technik. 1983;**55**(4):322-323. DOI: 10.1002/cite.330550422

[44] Wagner B. Leistungsvergleich von Bioreaktoren für mycelförmiges Wachstum [thesis]. Zurich: ETH Zurich; 1987. DOI: 10.3929/ethz-a-000412561

[45] Monk JM, Koza A, Campodonico MA, Machado D, Seoane JM, Palsson BO, et al. Multi-omics quantification of species variation of *Escherichia coli* links molecular features with strain phenotypes. Cell Systems. 2016 Sep;**3**(3):238-251. DOI: 10.1016/j.cels.2016.08.013

[46] Schneider E. Die Prokaryonta und die prokaryontische Zelle. In: Fuchs G, Schlegel HG, editors. Allgemeine Mikrobiologie. 8th ed. Stuttgart: Georg Thieme Verlag; 2007. pp. 31-56

[47] Schöb R. Centrifugal pump without bearings or seals. World Pumps. 2002 Jul;**2002**(430):34-37. DOI: 10.1016/S0262-1762(02)80218-8

[48] Wang F, Zheng Q, Wang B. Torque and levitation force comparison of bearingless motor with different rotor structures. In: ICEMS'2001 Proceedings of the Fifth International Conference on Electrical Machines and Systems (IEEE Cat No01EX501); Int. Acad. Publishers. pp. 1057-1060. DOI: 10.1109/ICEMS.2001.971860

[49] Shih T-H, Liou WW, Shabbir A, Yang Z, Zhu J. A new k-ϵ eddy viscosity model for high Reynolds number turbulent flows. Computers and Fluids. 1995 Mar;**24**(3):227-238. DOI: 10.1016/0045-7930(94)00032-T

[50] Biener R, Steinkämper A, Hofmann J. Calorimetric control for high cell density cultivation of a recombinant *Escherichia coli* strain. Journal of Biotechnology. 2010 Mar;**146**(1-2):45-53. DOI: 10.1016/j.jbiotec.2010.01.004

[51] Riesenberg D, Schulz V, Knorre WA, Pohl H, Korz D, Sanders E, et al. High cell density cultivation of *Escherichia coli* at controlled specific growth rate. Journal of Biotechnology. 1991 Aug;**20**(1):17-27. DOI: 10.1016/0168-1656(91)90032-Q

[52] Lee SY. High cell-density culture of *Escherichia coli*. Trends in Biotechnology. 1996 Mar;**14**(3):98-105. DOI: 10.1016/0167-7799(96)80930-9

[53] Lara AR, Galindo E, Ramírez OT, Palomares LA. Living with heterogeneities in bioreactors: Understanding the effects of environmental gradients on cells. Molecular Biotechnology. 2006 Dec;**34**(3):355-382. DOI: 10.1385/MB:34:3:355

[54] Zlokarnik M. Rührtechnik. Berlin, Heidelberg: Springer Berlin Heidelberg; 1999. 347 p. DOI: 10.1007/978-3-642-58635-4

[55] Jensen EB, Carlsen S. Production of recombinant human growth hormone in *Escherichia coli*: Expression of different precursors and physiological effects of glucose, acetate, and salts. Biotechnology and Bioengineering. 1990 Jun 5;**36**(1):1-11. DOI: 10.1002/bit.260360102

[56] Pan JG, Rhee JS, Lebeault JM. Physiological constraints in increasing biomass concentration of *Escherichia coli* b in fed-batch culture. Biotechnology Letters. 1987 Feb;**9**(2):89-94. DOI: 10.1007/BF01032744

[57] Xu B, Jahic M, Enfors S-O. Modeling of overflow metabolism in batch and fed-batch cultures of *Escherichia coli*. Biotechnology Progress. 1999 Feb 5;**15**(1):81-90. DOI: 10.1021/bp9801087

[58] Shiloach J, Fass R. Growing *E. coli* to high cell density—A historical perspective on method development. Biotechnology Advances. 2005 Jul;**23**(5):345-357. DOI: 10.1016/j.biotechadv.2005.04.004

[59] Kaiser SC, Perepelitsa N, Dittler I, Eibl D. Experiences with a benchtop-scale glass bioreactor: Engineering data and cultivation results. Bioprocess International. 2015;**13**(10):46-52

[60] Kaiser SC, Eibl R, Eibl D. Engineering characteristics of a single-use stirred bioreactor at bench-scale: The Mobius CellReady 3L bioreactor as a case study. Engineering in Life Sciences. 2011;**11**(4):359-368. DOI: 10.1002/elsc.201000171

[61] Eppendorf AG. Parallel CHO cell cultivation in Eppendorf BioBLU ® c single-use bioreactors. Application Note No. 355. 2017

[62] Sartorius Stedim Biotech GmbH. CHO cell-based production of a secreted model protein using the novel BIOSTAT ® A. Application Note #08. 2015

[63] Kaiser SC, Blaschczok K, Eibl D. Novel CHO suspension cell cultivation. Genetic Engineering & Biotechnology News. 2013;**33**(14):32-33. DOI: 10.1089/gen.33.14.17

[64] Kaiser SC, Blaschczok K, Eibl D. Cultivation of CHO suspension cells and seap expression in the finesse glass bioreactor. In: Industry Yearbook 2015-2016. Boston: BioProcess International; 2015. p. 30

[65] Eibl R, Kaiser SC, Lombriser R, Eibl D. Disposable bioreactors: The current state-of-the-art and recommended applications in biotechnology. Applied Microbiology and Biotechnology. 2010 Mar;**86**(1):41-49. DOI: 10.1007/s00253-009-2422-9

[66] Eibl R, Löffelholz C, Eibl D. Disposable bioreactors for inoculum production and protein expression. In: Pörtner R, editor. Animal Cell Biotechnology. Methods in Molecular

Biology (Methods and Protocols). Totowa, NJ: Humana Press; 2014. pp. 265-284. DOI: 10.1007/978-1-62703-733-4_18

[67] Eppendorf AG. Scale-up of *Escherichia coli* fermentation from small scale to pilot scale using Eppendorf fermentation systems. Application Note No. 306; 2016

[68] Maier B, Dietrich C, Büchs J. Correct application of the sulphite oxidation methodology of measuring the volumetric mass transfer coefficient k_La under non-pressurized and pressurized conditions. Food and Bioproducts Processing: Transactions of the Institution of Chemical Engineers, Part C. 2001;**79**(2):107-113. DOI: 10.1205/096030801750286267

[69] Junker BH. Scale-up methodologies for *Escherichia coli* and yeast fermentation processes. Journal of Bioscience and Bioengineering. 2004;**97**(6):347-364. DOI: 10.1263/jbb.97.347

[70] Sartorius Stedim Biotech GmbH. High-cell-density cultivation of *Escherichia coli* in a BIOSTAT ® D-DCU 10-3 Stainless Steel Bioreactor. Application Note #06; 2013

[71] Dreher T, Walcarius B, Husemann U, Klingenberg F, Zahnow C, Adams T, et al. Microbial high cell density fermentations in a stirred single-use bioreactor. In: Eibl D, Eibl R, editors. Disposable Bioreactors II. Berlin, Heidelberg: Springer Berlin Heidelberg; 2013. pp. 127-147. DOI: 10.1007/10_2013_189

[72] Jones N. Single-use processing for microbial fermentations. Bioprocess International. 2015;**13**(4):56-62

[73] Knoll A, Bartsch S, Husemann B, Engel P, Schroer K, Ribeiro B, et al. High cell density cultivation of recombinant yeasts and bacteria under non-pressurized and pressurized conditions in stirred tank bioreactors. Journal of Biotechnology. 2007;**132**(2):167-179. DOI: 10.1016/j.jbiotec.2007.06.010

[74] Eppendorf AG. A comparative study: Small scale *E. coli* cultivation using BioBLU ® single-use and reusable vessels. Application Note No. 297; 2014

[75] GE Healthcare. Microbial fermentation in single-use Xcellerex XDR-50 MO fermentor system. Application Note 29-0564-39 AB; 2014

Section 6

Regulation

Chapter 6

Scientific and Regulatory Perspective on Monoclonal Antibody Biosimilars

Po-Chih Wu, Yi-Chen Yang, Der-Yuan Wang and
Hwei-Fang Cheng

Additional information is available at the end of the chapter

http://dx.doi.org/10.5772/intechopen.78583

Abstract

Similar biotherapeutic products (SBPs), also called biosimilars, exhibit similar biological and clinical properties to authorized reference products. Biosimilars, including small molecules like erythropoietin and complex macromolecules like monoclonal antibodies (mAbs), have been used extensively in disease treatment. Monoclonal antibody biosimilars have gradually become a dominant development in the global pharmaceutical industry since their patents or data protection have been expired or nearing expiration. Since the mAb biosimilars are complex biological macromolecules with various post-translation modifications, it is important to evaluate whether these tiny differences significantly affect the quality. From a regulatory perspective, the comparability study needs to be performed to demonstrate that the quality, safety, and efficacy are similar to the biological reference. Based on these comprehensive comparative results, the indicated extrapolation might be acceptable. Post-market surveillance is also required because of unexpected biological variation caused by slightly different manufacturing processes. This chapter presents the scientific and regulatory considerations for monoclonal antibody biosimilar products for manufactures and for the regulatory authorities to administrate wisely and comprehensively.

Keywords: biosimilar, monoclonal antibody, biosimilar monoclonal antibody, regulatory perspective, comparability study

1. Introduction

The developments of "copies" of drug products, such as generic drugs or biosimilars, have become the trend in the pharmaceutical markets. However, in fact, they are strikingly different in respect of the structure, developments, and approval requirements [1]. Unlike the generic drug, which is chemically synthesized, the biosimilar is a complex molecule with many post-translational modifications, because it is produced from the complex living cells. In contrast to the generic drug, the biosimilar has immunogenic potentials. Furthermore, only the bioequivalence study is required for the approval of generic drug products in the regulatory requirements; whereas, for biosimilar products, the comparative study to demonstrate the biosimilarity to reference products is required [2–4]. The biosimilar is a biological product, which exhibits high similarities to the products already licensed in terms of quality, safety, and efficacy. However, the exact definition of "biosimilar" itself does not reach the consensus among different regulatory agencies [5]. Despite these differences among regions, the basic principles for biosimilars are similar [6, 7]. For harmonization on the evaluation and regulation of biosimilars, the guideline on the evaluation of similar biotherapeutic products (SBPs) is provided by WHO Expert Committee on Biological Standardization (ECBS) [8].

Monoclonal antibodies (mAbs) are the fastest growing class of biotherapeutic products for treating cancer or inflammatory diseases and they can be found on the lists of the top 10 global annual pharmaceutical revenues. As the patents or data protections have been expired or nearing expiration, many global pharmaceutical industries have turned toward developing similar mAb biotherapeutic products. The similar mAb biotherapeutic products, also called biosimilar mAbs, exhibit highly similar biological and clinical properties to the authorized reference mAbs. The entry of these products into the markets could help to slow the increasing healthcare costs due to its affordability and accessibility. The mAb is a complex macromolecule with several sizes and charge variants or post-translational modifications, including different glycosylation profiles, or N and C terminal heterogeneities. The presence of differences is shown in each mAb due to the structural complexity. Although these differences are seemingly tiny, it is possible to have large impacts on the quality of final products. Therefore, additional guidelines that apply to mAb-derived products are demanding. In 2016, WHO guideline on the evaluation of biosimilar mAb products was adopted by the ECBS [9]. The document provides some critical considerations for manufactures as well as regulatory authorities for characterizing or assessing the quality of biosimilar mAb products. However, until now, there have been no standard analytical methods or clear specifications for defining the similarity in the nonclinical and clinical comparability studies. The manufactures have to develop their own analytical methods to prove similarity in relation to reference products, and these analytical methods are required to be scientifically validated [10].

The quality attributes of biosimilar mAb products might be affected by the manufacturing process. Manufacturers of biosimilar mAbs do not easily obtain the detailed information about the manufacturing process of the reference products or the usage of the active ingredients [11]. In general, the amino acid sequence of the biosimilar mAbs must be identical to the reference mAbs; however, other characteristics, including the structure conformation, biological activity, or contents of impurities, might vary from products to products. To obtain the approval from the regulatory authorities, the comparability studies of structural and functional characterization and process-derived impurities of the biosimilar products and reference products are required [12]. Moreover, one mAb biotherapeutic product might apply to multiple indications and exert the clinical effects through different mechanisms of action (MoA) [13]. Therefore, the comparability studies in the clinical trials are also required. If any clinical differences of biosimilar mAbs compared to reference mAbs are found, additional evaluations must be justified to exclude any adverse effects [14]. However, there are many challenges for developing biosimilar mAbs, including the harmonization of analytical methods, development of comparative assay, and exact definitions of biological activity in the clinical trials [15]. Due to the complexity of bioprocess in the biosimilar mAbs, very tiny differences in the manufacturing process might have large impacts on the quality of final products. The development process and critical concerns in each step are described as follows, which would be helpful for manufactures as well as regulatory authorities to administrate with more scientific and regulatory considerations.

2. Framework of development

From the point of product approval, the development of biosimilar mAbs may be divided into the pre-market and post-market stage. In the pre-market stage, to obtain the approval from the regulatory agencies, the biosimilar mAbs must undergo a rigorous development process and comparative study to demonstrate the quality, safety, and efficacy similarity to the reference mAbs. After the product approval, in order to achieve the maximal safety and quality of mAb biosimilar products, post-market surveillance is indispensable. The framework of biosimilar mAb development and critical points for considerations are shown in **Figure 1** [16].

2.1. Manufacturing development

Biosimilar mAbs are developed to show similarity to reference mAbs in terms of quality, safety, and efficacy. The manufacturing development of biosimilar mAb products might be different from that of reference mAbs, because some detailed information of the manufacturing process of reference mAb is not accessible by the manufactures [11]. In order to reduce any unnecessary clinical safety and efficacy effects, the manufacturing process should be optimized to minimize the differences between biosimilar mAbs and reference mAbs. It is advisable that the manufacturing process of biosimilar mAbs should be as similar as possible to that of reference mAbs and the manufactures should understand each manufacturing process. If any differences in the manufacturing process are found, the potential impacts of changing elements on the product quality, safety, and efficacy should be evaluated and justified [17].

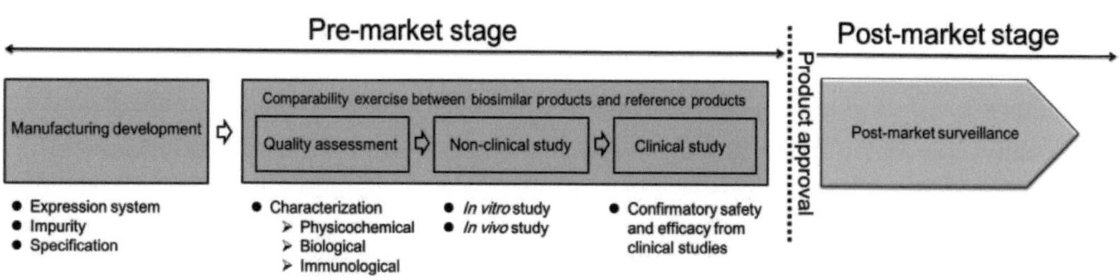

Figure 1. Framework development and critical points for considerations of biosimilar mAbs.

2.1.1. Expression system

Choice of suitable expression system is one of the critical points for the manufacturing process. According to the WHO guidelines, a different expression system is allowed for the production of biosimilar mAb products [8, 9]. Although the primary structure (amino acid sequence) is not affected by different host cell lines, the protein modifications, including N-terminal truncation, C-terminal truncation, or post-translation modification, and process-derived impurities like residual host DNAs or residual host proteins might be affected. These changes might indirectly affect the biological effects in the clinical consequences. In most cases, when different host cell types are used, different glycosylation profiles might be found [18]. For example, the mAb products produced from mouse cell lines, like NS0 or SP2/0 cells, have alpha-1,3-gal in their carbohydrate structure. However, there is no production of such structure in the human cell lines, because these cell lines lack the necessary enzyme to synthesize the alpha-1,3-gal antigens [19]. Moreover, the immune response against this"special" glycosylation structure would be triggered in the human body, which might lead to the adverse clinical effects. This situation could be avoided by using Chinese hamster ovary (CHO) cells [20]. Therefore, to minimize the differences between biosimilar products and reference products, the choice of the expression system for the mAb biosimilar products should be carefully considered. In general, it is advisable for the manufactures to choose the same host cell type as that of reference mAbs to minimize the possible impact on the clinical efficacy and safety of the products when developing mAb biosimilars.

2.1.2. Impurity

Product impurity is inevitable in the manufacturing process. Impurities, the components which are not desired in the drug substance or drug products, might trigger some safety concerns [21]. To ensure the safety of products, the differences of impurity profiles between the biosimilar mAbs and reference mAbs need to be evaluated. For mAb products, the testing of impurity includes the analysis of residual host DNA, residual protein A, or monomer contents in the products. If any differences between biosimilar mAbs and reference mAbs are significantly observed, additional evaluation of the impurity-derived impacts on the product safety and efficacy is required [8, 12, 22].

2.1.3. Specification

The specification (acceptance criteria) needs to be considered in the manufacturing process. The specification of biosimilar mAbs is not actually the same as that of reference mAbs. Sufficient batches of biosimilar mAb products are needed for the collaborative study. The setting of specification of biosimilar mAbs is based on the manufacturing experiences or comparative results of the collaborative study on biosimilar mAbs and reference mAbs. In general, the limit setting of biosimilar mAbs should not be wider than the range of variability of reference mAbs. If the acceptance criteria of biosimilar mAbs are significantly out of the acceptable range of reference mAbs, additional evidence to confirm the safety of products is needed [21, 23].

2.2. Comparability exercise

From the regulatory requirements, the comparability exercise of biosimilar mAbs and reference mAbs must be needed. According to ICH Q5E, the comparability study should prove that the proposed product is highly similar to the reference product before and after the manufacturing process changes [24]. The comparability data of quality attributes might be the foundation for reducing the requirements of non-clinical and clinical studies. When considering that batch variabilities might affect the results of comparability exercise, products from different batches should be evaluated. What is more, the analytical methods in the comparability exercise should be sensitive to detect the potential differences between biosimilar mAbs and reference mAbs and the parameter ranges for each analytical methods need to be determined by an appropriate statistical analysis [8, 9, 25].

To obtain representative data from the comparability exercise, the choice of a suitable reference mAb is important. Comprehensive information of reference mAbs could be the foundation for the establishment of quality, safety, and efficacy profiles, to which are the biosimilar mAbs compared. Head-to-head comparisons are performed to demonstrate high level of biosimilarity between the biosimilar mAbs and reference mAbs in the comparability exercise [26]. Following considerations are provided for the choice of suitable reference mAb biotherapeutic products [8, 12, 22].

- Whether the reference products have already been authorized based on the integrated set of quality, safety, and efficacy data.
- Whether the drug substance, active ingredient, and the biological function of biosimilar mAbs are similar to those of reference mAbs.
- Whether the dosage form and route of administration of biosimilar mAbs are identical to that of reference mAbs.
- Whether the same reference products are used throughout the comparative quality, safety, and efficacy studies.

2.2.1. Quality assessment

The quality comparative studies are conducted by the state-of-art analytical techniques and appropriate analytical methods. The analytical methods should be sensitive enough to detect any differences between biosimilar mAbs and reference mAbs. For the development of analytical methods, the information of the analytical limitations, like specificity in each analytical technique should be known by the manufactures. The characteristics including physicochemical, biological, and other related properties (e.g., impurities, finished products, and specification) are analyzed by the head-to-head comparative studies [27–30]. For mAb analysis, the common characteristics and analytical methods to ensure product quality are provided in **Table 1**, and these analytical items could also be applied to the comparative study of biosimilar mAbs and reference mAbs [5].

Characteristics	Items	Analytical methods
Primary structure	Intact mass analysis	Mass spectrometric analysis
	Peptide mapping	Enzyme digestion and HPLC
	N-terminal sequence	Edman degradation
	C-terminal sequence	Peptide mapping and intact molecular mass analysis
	Disulfide bond bridge analysis	Peptide mapping under nonreduced condition
	Glycosylation site	Peptide mapping with mass spectrometric analysis
Higher order structure	Structure analysis	Circular dichroism
Post-translational modification	Glycan profiles	Enzyme digestion and mass spectrometric analysis
	Sialic acid content	HPAEC-PAD
Heterogeneity	Isoforms	cIEF
Immunological activity	Binding affinity	Enzyme immunoassay
Biological activity	Potency	Cell-based assay
Purity/impurity	Product-related impurity	HPLC
Process-related impurity	Host cell protein	ELISA
	Residual DNA	PCR
	Residual protein A	ELISA
	Endotoxin	LAL

HPAEC-PAD: high performance anion exchange chromatography with pulsed amperometric detection; HPLC: high-performance liquid chromatography; cIEF: capillary isoelectric focusing; ELISA: enzyme-linked immunosorbent assay; PCR: polymerase chain reaction; LAL: limulus amebocyte lysate.

Table 1. Analytical items and analytical methods for the analysis of mAb characterization.

2.2.1.1. Physicochemical properties

The characterization of physicochemical properties for biosimilar mAbs is required, due to the inherent complexity of mAb products. The monoclonal antibody is a macromolecule with size and charge variants and different post-translational modifications. The structural heterogeneity should be analyzed by the state-of art techniques. The physicochemical testing should include the determination of the primary structure (e.g., amino acid sequence), higher order structure (e.g., disulfide bond bridges, free thiol functional group, and secondary or tertiary structures), and some physicochemical properties (e.g., charge variants, site-specific glycosylation patterns, or glycan profiles) [12].

The analysis of the primary structure is the determination of the amino acid sequence of products. In general, the primary structure of mAb SBPs should be identical to that of reference mAbs, except for the structural heterogeneity in the N-terminus or C-terminus. Peptide mapping is a common analytical method to identify or quantify the abundance of heterogeneous forms. For higher order structures, the conformation stability is critical for functional properties. For example, the differences in intra-disulfide bridges could directly affect the IgG2 affinities in mAb products [31]. The commonly analytical techniques used in the testing include hydrogen-deuterium exchange mass spectrometry (H/DX-MS), circular dichroism (CD), and two-dimensional nuclear magnetic resonance (2D-NMR). H/DX-MS is used to identify the rigid or flexible domain of the protein structure in the formulation conditions, CD is used to assess the content of secondary structure, and 2D-NMR is used to analyze the integrity of protein structure [32]. In some situations, a combination of two or more analytical techniques, like capillary electrophoresis coupled with mass spectrometry, might be powerful in characterizing the physicochemical properties [33].

The comparability exercise on the post-translational modification of biosimilar mAbs and reference mAbs is required in the physicochemical analysis. The comparative glycan analysis includes the N-glycan analysis, site-specific glycosylation patterns, or overall glycan profile [34]. Given that small differences in glycan profiles could cause unexpectedly immunogenic consequences, additional data to support the product safety are required. Moreover, the high heterogeneity of the active ingredients increases the complexity of the structure or other physicochemical properties, which caused it difficult to analyze the different variants in one analytical method. To solve these problems, the combination of the different analytical methods, like ion exchange chromatography, isoelectric focusing, and capillary electrophoresis, is developed. However, the analytical techniques of physicochemical analytical methods are restricted to its detection limits, so that some higher order structure of the molecule or slight difference of mAb SBPs and reference mAbs are not easily detected by the physicochemical analysis. To complement the detection limits of physicochemical analysis, the biological analysis is performed to determine whether the heterogeneous variants have impact on the product safety.

2.2.1.2. Biological activity properties

Biological activity, also called potency, is defined as the product's specific ability to achieve the intended biological effects. It is an important parameter for characterizing the product quality and batch analysis. Biological assay is the quantitative measure of the biological activity and reflects the mechanism of action of the functional protein. The data obtained from the biological assays could connect to the clinical activity. Additionally, the biological assay complements the physicochemical analysis to confirm the structural integrity of the molecules. The analytical method for biological activity should be specific and sensitive enough to detect slight differences in batch analysis or comparative study. The biological activity should be determined by calibrating against international or national standards, and the results could be expressed in international units (IU) or units (U) of activity [8, 9, 12].

The mechanism of the action of mAbs varies ranging from simple antigen binding, which alone affects the clinical response, to antigen binding with one or more immunological effects, which combines to present an overall clinical response. For example, infliximab, which is a chimeric monoclonal antibody specific for tumor necrosis factor alpha (TNF-α), achieves clinical efficacy in rheumatoid arthritis through the mechanism of antigen binding [35]. However, rituximab, specific for binding to CD20, requires the Fc function for its clinical efficacy in all the clinical indications [36]. The mAb consists of two major functional domains, including Fab and Fc fragments. For characterizing biological activity properties, the assay should be designed for analyzing binding affinity and functional activities of these two regions. If it can be shown that the clinical effects are only affected through antigen binding, the ligand binding assays could estimate biological activity. Given that the Fc part of mAb might mediate the immunobiological effects, the relevant, validated potency assay for the determination of other immunobiological effects other than just potency should be developed. In this regard, the choice of appropriate cell-based assays to determine the potency should be considered.

2.2.1.3. Immunological properties (immunogenicity)

Immunogenicity is the ability/capability of molecules to elicit the immune response against external substances. The immune response against the mAb biotherapeutic products is affected by many factors, including the drug substances, excipients, process derived impurities, route of administration, dosing regimen, or other related factors [12]. For the analysis of immunological properties, the binding specificity, binding affinity, and binding kinetics all need to be analyzed by scientifically analytical methods, such as surface plasmon response, microcalorimetry, or classical Scatchard analysis. Moreover, the Fab-associated functions (neutralization of soluble antigens or receptor activation/blockade) and the Fc-associated functions (antibody-dependent cell cytotoxicity, complement-dependent cell cytotoxicity, apoptosis, or complement activation) should also be analyzed using appropriate analytical methods [8, 9]. These analytical methods should be sensitive enough to detect the difference between biosimilar products and reference products.

2.2.2. Nonclinical study

Nonclinical study encompasses the pharmacological/toxicological assessments of biosimilar products. By referring to the results from the physicochemical and biological characterization studies, the nonclinical study program is designed to detect potential impacts on safety and efficacy of biosimilar products. Nonclinical studies can be divided into *in vitro* studies and *in vivo* studies. *In vitro* studies should be conducted first, since the results from *in vitro* studies could make a decision to the extent of what *in vivo* studies are required. The considerations for *in vitro* studies and *in vivo* studies are discussed as follows [9, 37, 38].

2.2.2.1. In vitro study

To assess the difference of biological activity between a biosimilar product and a reference product, *in vitro* studies should be performed. Compared to animal studies, an *in vitro* assay is more specific and sensitive to detect differences between the biosimilar products and reference products [39]. For establishments of *in vitro* studies of biosimilar mAbs, the following points should be taken into account.

- The assay needs to be scientifically valid and has the ability to detect biological differences between biosimilar mAbs and reference mAbs, not just the response of biosimilar mAbs.
- An appropriate number of batches of reference mAbs and biosimilar mAbs are required, given that the results will be affected by variabilities with different batches.
- The number of tests should be adjusted sufficiently to make the meaningful conclusions that biosimilar mAbs demonstrate similarity in biological activity to reference mAbs.
- The data from *in vitro* studies should cover the pharmacological/toxicological assessments, which could be a reference supportive for the clinical design.

For nonclinical *in vitro* program of biosimilar mAbs, the biological analysis of Fab and Fc fragments should be included. Following table summarizes the analytical items and analytical methods in the nonclinical *in vitro* program of biosimilar mAbs [9] (**Table 2**).

2.2.2.2. *In vivo study*

In vivo study is designed to provide more information on "unexpected" pharmacological/toxicological activities relevant to the clinical application. Such studies could be comparative in nature and can detect the differences between biosimilar products and reference products. However, when the necessary information has already obtained from *in vitro* studies, *in vivo* studies are not required. Following points are provided for the determination of the need for *in vivo* studies [40].

	Item		**Method**
	Fab-associated	**Fc-associated**	
Binding studies	• Target antigen binding	• Binding to Fc receptors (FcγRI, FcγRII, FcγRIII, and FcRn) • Binding to complement (C1q)	• ELISA • Surface plasmon resonance (SPR) • Flow cytometry
Biological activities/ functional assay	• Neutralization of soluble ligand • Receptor activation • Receptor blockade	• Antibody-dependent cell cytotoxicity (ADCC) • Complement-dependent cytotoxicity (CDC) • Complement activation • Apoptosis	• Cell-based assay

Table 2. Analytical items and analytical methods of ***in vitro*** nonclinical study of biosimilar mAbs.

- The data of biological activity or pharmacodynamics could be available from the biological assays in the part of the quality assessment. If these data are sufficiently reliable to reflect the relevant clinical situation, *in vivo* studies would not be necessary. Accordingly, if the data are not fully elucidated by *in vitro* assay, *in vivo* assay is required.
- The monoclonal antibodies might mediate the unprecedented effects that cannot be fully characterized by an *in vitro* assay. In this situation, *in vivo* studies are required to provide complementary information.

If *in vivo* studies are required, the following points are needed for consideration.

- Choice of animal species and the relevant models (in-breed animals, transgenic animals, or transplant models) for the assay.
- If there are no appropriate animal models for *in vivo* assay, the manufacture needs to evaluate any potential risks by the data from *in vitro* assay, when proceeding to the clinical trials.
- Some factors need to be considered, when considering whether the additional *in vivo* assays should be performed

  1. Presence of potential quality attributes in biosimilar mAb products, which have not been detected in the reference mAbs.
  2. The relevant quantitative differences in the comparative measurements between biosimilar mAbs and reference mAbs.
  3. The difference formulation is used. For example, the excipient is not commonly used in the mAbs.

2.2.3. Clinical study

Clinical study for biosimilar mAb aims to confirm the safety and efficacy issues from the clinical view. For the design in the biosimilar mAb clinical trial program, the natural characteristics, intended indication, and duration should be taken into consideration. In fact, the design of most comparative clinical study is based on the clinical experiences, which had already been acquired from the reference mAb. It is advisable to use the finished products for clinical studies, so as to obtain pivotal data for marketing authorization from the regulatory authorities. The clinical comparability exercise is performed in a step-wise procedure, and usually begins with the clinical pharmacodynamics (PD) and pharmacokinetic (PK) studies, followed by the comparative clinical safety and efficacy study in a selected indication. Due to the clinical experiences of reference products, some steps of the biosimilar mAb clinical trial are not necessary, such that the phase 2 clinical trial (dose finding study) is not required, when the dosage used in the biosimilar mAb administration regimen is the same as that used in the reference mAb [11, 41]. Therefore, compared to the development of reference mAbs, the development of biosimilar mAbs needs less time.

The extent and number of clinical trials of biosimilar mAbs compared to reference mAbs could be affected by the following factors [42]:

- The intrinsic complexity (structural and biological properties) of biosimilar mAbs.
- The limitations of studies in the nonclinical comparative structural and biological study.

- The complexity of mechanisms of action of biosimilar mAbs.
- The degree of uncertainty of biosimilar mAbs in efficacy and safety issues.
- The clinical experiences obtained from the reference mAbs.

Although the clinical trial design of biosimilar mAbs followed the same guideline as other similar biotherapeutic products, additional considerations are required. The indication extrapolation is one of the important considerations for biosimilar mAb clinical studies. To provide justification for indication extrapolation, the equivalence clinical trial is preferred over the noninferiority trial. An equivalence trial is demonstrated to confirm that the biosimilar mAb is clinically similar to the reference mAb. This demonstration could provide the efficacy and safety data of biosimilar mAbs that could be a strong rationale for extrapolation to other indications of reference mAbs. In an equivalence trail, it is advisable to choose the sensitive and well-established study models regarding to the study population and study endpoints, given that assay with sensitivity should have the ability to detect differences between the biosimilar mAbs and reference mAbs, even if only tiny difference exists. In order to minimize the impacts on inter-patients variability, the selected study population for the clinical trial should be homogeneous and increase the likelihood that the observed clinical effects are caused by the difference between biosimilar mAbs and reference mAbs. In general, patients without previous treatments are good study models, because the observed clinical effects could exclude the interference effects of other medications [42–45].

2.3. Post-market surveillance

Post-market surveillance is an important process in achieving a maximum safety and effectiveness of mAb biosimilars. It is a long-term monitoring to detect or assess any product-derived adverse effects. Some of these effects may not easily be detected during the preapproval clinical testing, because the narrow population is tested in the trials. In addition, due to the changes of material sources, facility or regulatory requirements, the manufacturing process of biosimilar mAb products might change. In some situations, the profiles of post-translational modification alter during the product life cycle, which might directly or indirectly affect the product safety or effectiveness. For example, Remicade (infliximab) has gone through over 35 changes since product approval in 1999, but no any adverse effects were reported in the clinical usage [46]. However, the change of glycosylation profiles of Rituxan (anti-CD20 antibody) has been reported from batches to batches, which directly or indirectly affects the product immunogenicity [47]. Therefore, continuous post-marketing surveillance of products is required so as to make prompt prevention for adverse effects.

The following considerations are indicated when designing the program of post-marketing safety monitoring.

- Whether to identify low-frequency adverse reactions associated with biosimilar mAb products (not easy to identify the pre-marketing stages).
- Whether to identify some high-risk groups.
- Whether to discern that the adverse effects are caused by the biosimilar mAb product, not by the reference mAb.

- Whether safety monitoring is continuous.
- Whether the risk or hazard prevention measures could be initiated promptly.

3. Indication extrapolation

The comparative study data of biosimilar products and reference products in one indication could extrapolate to other indications, in which reference products originally have been approved. Extrapolation is an important process for biosimilar developments, because it could reduce/eliminate the need for duplicative clinical studies [48]. The recommended principles of indication extrapolation of biosimilar mAbs could refer to the WHO guidance document about the evaluation of SBP. In general, to make indication extrapolation possible, the following points are needed.

- The mechanism of action of a biosimilar product and a reference product is the same.
- The clinical test is sensitive enough to detect the potential differences between biosimilar products and reference products.
- The safety and immunogenicity data of biosimilar products in one indication are well characterized and there are no additional safety concerns when extrapolating these data to other indications.
- Additional convincing data must be provided to support extrapolation to other conditions of use.

For biosimilar mAbs, some points should be considered. Unlike other biologics, monoclonal antibodies have two functional domain—Fab and Fc domains. Each domain might exert their clinical effects through different mechanisms, including the receptor blockage, signaling induction or down-regulation, receptor down-regulation, and cell cytotoxicity (ADCC, CDC, or apoptosis). One monoclonal antibody might exert the clinical effects through one or a combination of these mechanisms in different indications. For example, infliximab does not require Fc function in rheumatologic and psoriatic indications; however, it exerts the clinical effects through the Fc domain in inflammatory bowel disease (IBD) [49]. When the mechanism of action (MoA) of biosimilar products is different to that of reference products, the indication extrapolation could be challenging. In some cases, the drug dosage of one product might not be the same between different indications; therefore, different dosages are needed to be tested. Moreover, a reference mAb might hold different types of indications. For example, rituximab (anti-CD20 mAb) is authorized for the treatment of both inflammatory diseases and cancer [50]. Since the pharmacokinetic data are different between these two diseases, it is inappropriate for biosimilar products to extrapolate.

4. Conclusions

With the trend of global pharmaceutical developments, the era of biosimilar mAbs has begun. It is clear that the entry of biosimilar products to the markets would bring benefits for science and healthcare. With regard to biosimilar mAb manufactures, the reduction of production costs, choice of suitable cells, and control parameters setting to avoid product heterogeneity are important in the manufacturing process. From the regulatory perspective, the abbreviated development program is adopted in the biosimilar mAb products. Besides the data, which support the quality, safety, and efficacy of products, the comparative data to demonstrate the similarity between the biosimilar mAb product and the reference product needed to be submitted. Considering the impacts of batch variability on comparative results, different lots of products should be included in the in-depth comparative analysis. The integrated set of data from the comparative results would be the foundation for biosimilar development and the determination of the need for the extents that animal studies and clinical trials should be performed. For the clinical studies, it is advisable to choose one condition of use that would be sensitive to detect the clinical meaningful differences between the proposed biosimilar mAb and the reference mAb. However, some product-derived adverse effects might not be easily detected during the preapproval clinical testing. Based on the regulatory guideline requirements, pharmacovigilance and risk management plan for biosimilar mAbs should be submitted to regulatory authorities for dossier review. The risk management plans, which are proposed by the manufactures, should include the detailed information on the safety and risk concerns. However, challenges remain with an abbreviated pathway for biosimilar mAbs, including the lack of detailed information and acceptance criteria for biosimilarity demonstration. In order to promote the global development and achieve the maximal safety of biosimilar mAbs, it is expected that manufacturers should cooperate with regulatory authorities to fight against current challenges with more detailed scientific considerations from a regulatory perspective.

Author details

Po-Chih Wu, Yi-Chen Yang, Der-Yuan Wang and Hwei-Fang Cheng*

*Address all correspondence to: rmhfcheng@fda.gov.tw

Taiwan Food and Drug Administration, Taipei City, Taiwan

References

[1] van de Vooren K, Curto A, Garattini L. Biosimilar versus generic drugs: Same but different? Applied Health Economics and Health Policy. 2015;**13**(2):125-127. DOI: 10.1007/s40258-015-0154-9

[2] Camacho LH, Frost CP, Abella E, Morrow PK, Whittaker S. Biosimilars 101: Considerations for U.S. oncologists in clinical practice. Cancer Medicine. 2014;**3**(4):889-899. DOI: 10.1002/cam4.258

[3] Niederwieser D, Schmitz S. Biosimilar agents in oncology/haematology: From approval to practice. European Journal of Haematology. 2011;**86**(4):277-288. DOI: 10.1111/j.1600-0609.2010.01566.x

[4] Declerck P, Danesi R, Petersel D, Jacobs I. The Language of biosimilars: Clarification, definitions and regulatory aspects. Drugs. 2017;**77**(6):671-677. DOI: 10.1007/s40265-017-0717-1

[5] Tsuruta LR, Lopes dos Santos M, Moro AM. Biosimilars advancements: Moving on to the future, 49. Biotechnology Progress. 2015;**31**(5):1139. DOI: 10.1002/btpr.2066

[6] Wang J, Chow SC. On the regulatory approval pathway of biosimilar products. Pharmaceuticals. 2012;**5**(4):353-368. DOI: 10.3390/ph5040353

[7] Chugh PK, Roy V. Biosimilars: Current scientific and regulatory considerations. Current Clinical Pharmacology. 2014;**9**(1):53-63. DOI: 10.2174/15748847113089990066

[8] Guidelines on evaluation of similar biotherapeutic products (SBPs). In: WHO Expert Committee on Biological Standardization: Sixtieth report. Geneva: World Health Organization; 2013: Annex 2. Available from: http://apps.who.int/medicinedocs/documents/s19941en/s19941en.pdf

[9] Guidelines on evaluation of monoclonal antibodies as similar biotherapeutic products (SBPs). In: WHO Expert Committee on Biological Standardization: Sixty-fourth report. Geneva: World Health Organization; 2016: Annex 2. Available from: http://apps.who.int/medicinedocs/documents/s23321en/s23321en.pdf

[10] Hulse J, Cox C. *In vitro* functional testing methods for monoclonal antibody biosimilars. BioProcess International. 2013;**11**:24-27. Available from: http://www.bioprocessintl.com/manufacturing/monoclonal-antibodies/in-vitro-functional-testing-methods-for-monoclonal-antibody-biosimilars-344341/

[11] Weise M, Bielsky MC, De Smet K, Ehmann F, Ekman N, Narayanan G, et al. Biosimilars-why terminology matters. Nature Biotechnology. 2011;**29**(8):690-693. DOI: 10.1038/nbt.1936

[12] Guidance for industry. Quality Considerations in Demonstrating Biosimilarity of a Therapeutic Protein Product to a Reference Product. Silver Spring, MD: Food and Drug Administration; 2015. Available from: https://www.fda.gov/downloads/drugs/guidances/ucm291134.pdf

[13] Scott BJ, Klein AV, Wang J. Biosimilar monoclonal antibodies: A Canadian regulatory perspective on the assessment of clinically relevant differences and indication extrapolation. Journal of Clinical Pharmacology. 2015;**55**(Suppl 3):S123-S132. DOI: 10.1002/jcph.339

[14] Weise M, Bielsky MC, De Smet K, Ehmann F, Ekman N, Giezen TJ, et al. Biosimilars: What clinicians should know. Blood. 2012;**120**(26):5111-5117. DOI: 10.1182/blood-2012-04-425744

[15] McCamish M, Woollett G. Worldwide experience with biosimilar development. mAbs. 2011;**3**(2):209-217. DOI: 10.4161/mabs.3.2.15005

[16] McCamish M, Woollett G. The state of the art in the development of biosimilars. Clinical Pharmacology and Therapeutics. 2012;**91**(3):405-417. DOI: 10.1038/clpt.2011.343

[17] Reichert JM. Next generation and biosimilar monoclonal antibodies: Essential considerations towards regulatory acceptance in Europe. February 3-4, 2011, Freiburg, Germany. mAbs. 2011;**3**(3):223-240. DOI: 10.4161/mabs.3.3.15475

[18] Goh JB, Ng SK. Impact of host cell line choice on glycan profile. Critical Reviews in Biotechnology. 2017;**38**:1-17. DOI: 10.1080/07388551.2017.1416577

[19] Steinke JW, Platts-Mills TA, Commins SP. The alpha-gal story: Lessons learned from connecting the dots. The Journal of Allergy and Clinical Immunology. 2015;**135**(3):589-596. quiz 97. DOI: 10.1016/j.jaci.2014.12.1947

[20] Bosques CJ, Collins BE, Meador JW 3rd, Sarvaiya H, Murphy JL, Dellorusso G, et al. Chinese hamster ovary cells can produce galactose-alpha-1,3-galactose antigens on proteins. Nature Biotechnology. 2010;**28**(11):1153-1156. DOI: 10.1038/nbt1110-1153

[21] Preclinical safety evaluation of biotechnology-derived pharmaceuticals. ICH Guideline S6 (R1). Geneva, ICH Guideline Q5E. In: International Conference on Harmonisation of Technical Requirements for Registration of Pharmaceuticals for Human Use; 2011. Available from: http://www.ema.europa.eu/docs/ en_GB/document_library/Scientific_guideline/2009/09/WC500002828.pdf

[22] Guideline on Similar Biological Medicinal Products Containing Biotechnology-Derived Proteins as Active Substances: Quality Issues (Revision 1). European Medicines Agency; 2014. Available from: http://www.ema.europa.eu/docs/en_GB/document_library/Scientific_guideline/2014/06/WC500167838.pdf

[23] Specifications: Test procedures and acceptance criteria for biotechnological/biological products. ICH Guideline Q6B. In: International Conference on Harmonisation of Technical Requirements for Registration of Pharmaceuticals for Human Use; 1999. Available from: http://academy.gmp-compliance.org/guidemgr /files/3-1-17.pdf

[24] Comparability of biotechnological/biological products subject to changes in their manufacturing process. Geneva, ICH Guideline Q5E. In: International Conference on Harmonisation of Technical Requirements for Registration of Pharmaceuticals for Human Use; 2004. Available from: http://www.ich.org/fileadmin/Public_Web_Site/ICH_Products/Guidelines/Quality/Q5E/Step4/Q5E_Guideline.pdf

[25] Guideline on Comparability of Biotechnology-Derived Medicinal Products after Change in the Manufacturing Process. European Medicines Agency, London; 2007. Available from: http://www.ema.europa.eu/docs/en_GB/document_library/Scientific_guideline/2009/09/WC500003937.pdf

[26] Declerck P, Farouk Rezk M. The road from development to approval: Evaluating the body of evidence to confirm biosimilarity. Rheumatology. 2017;**56**(Suppl_4):iv4-iv13. DOI: 10.1093/rheumatology/kex279

[27] Jung SK, Lee KH, Jeon JW, Lee JW, Kwon BO, Kim YJ, et al. Physicochemical characterization of remsima. mAbs. 2014;**6**(5):1163-1177. DOI: 10.4161/mabs.32221

[28] Visser J, Feuerstein I, Stangler T, Schmiederer T, Fritsch C, Schiestl M. Physicochemical and functional comparability between the proposed biosimilar rituximab GP2013 and originator rituximab. BioDrugs: Clinical Immunotherapeutics, Biopharmaceuticals and Gene Therapy. 2013;**27**(5):495-507. DOI: 10.1007/s40259-013-0036-3

[29] Lopez-Morales CA, Miranda-Hernandez MP, Juarez-Bayardo LC, Ramirez-Ibanez ND, Romero-Diaz AJ, Pina-Lara N, et al. Physicochemical and biological characterization of a biosimilar trastuzumab. BioMed Research International. 2015;**2015**:427235. DOI: 10.1155/2015/427235

[30] Cho IH, Lee N, Song D, Jung SY, Bou-Assaf G, Sosic Z, et al. Evaluation of the structural, physicochemical, and biological characteristics of SB4, a biosimilar of etanercept. mAbs. 2016;**8**(6):1136-1155. DOI: 10.1080/19420862.2016.1193659

[31] Wei Z, Shacter E, Schenerman M, Dougherty J, McLeod LD. The role of higher-order structure in defining biopharmaceutical quality. BioProcess International. 2011;**9**:58-66. Available from: http://www.bioprocessintl.com/business/cmc-forums/the-role-of-higher-order-structure-in-defining-biopharmaceutical-quality-313472/

[32] Mielke SP, Krishnan VV. Characterization of protein secondary structure from NMR chemical shifts. Progress in Nuclear Magnetic Resonance Spectroscopy. 2009;**54** (3-4):141-165. DOI: 10.1016/j.pnmrs.2008.06.002

[33] Mischak H, Coon JJ, Novak J, Weissinger EM, Schanstra JP, Dominiczak AF. Capillary electrophoresis-mass spectrometry as a powerful tool in biomarker discovery and clinical diagnosis: An update of recent developments. Mass Spectrometry Reviews. 2009;**28**(5):703-724. DOI: 10.1002/mas.20205

[34] Zhang L, Luo S, Zhang B. Glycan analysis of therapeutic glycoproteins. mAbs. 2016;**8**(2):205-215. DOI: 10.1080/19420862.2015.1117719

[35] Maini RN, Feldmann M. How does infliximab work in rheumatoid arthritis? Arthritis Research. 2002;**4**(Suppl 2):S22-S28. DOI: 10.1186/ar549

[36] Boross P, Leusen JH. Mechanisms of action of CD20 antibodies. American Journal of Cancer Research. 2012;**2**(6):676-690. PMCID: PMC3512181

[37] Bui LA, Hurst S, Finch GL, Ingram B, Jacobs IA, Kirchhoff CF, et al. Key considerations in the preclinical development of biosimilars. Drug Discovery Today. 2015;**20**(Suppl 1): 3-15. DOI: 10.1016/j.drudis.2015.03.011

[38] Li EC, Abbas R, Jacobs IA, Yin D. Considerations in the early development of biosimilar products. Drug Discovery Today. 2015;**20**(Suppl 2):1-9. DOI: 10.1016/j.drudis.2014.12.017

[39] van Aerts LA, De Smet K, Reichmann G, van der Laan JW, Schneider CK. Biosimilars entering the clinic without animal studies. A paradigm shift in the European Union. mAbs. 2014;**6**(5):1155-1162. DOI: 10.4161/mabs.29848

[40] Guidance for Industry. Scientific Considerations in demonstrating biosimilartiy to a reference product. Silver Spring, MD: Food and Drug Administration; 2015. Available from: https://www.fda.gov/downloads/drugs/guidances/ucm291128.pdf

[41] Scotte F, Launay-Vacher V, Rey JB. Colony stimulating factors (CSF) biosimilars. Progress? Targeted Oncology. 2012;**7**(Suppl 1):S17-S24. DOI: 10.1007/s11523-011-0189-2

[42] Alten R, Cronstein BN. Clinical trial development for biosimilars. Seminars in Arthritis and Rheumatism. 2015;**44**(Suppl 6):S2-S8. DOI: 10.1016/j.semarthrit.2015.04.002

[43] Bui LA, Taylor C. Developing clinical trials for biosimilars. Seminars in Oncology. 2014;**41**(Suppl 1):S15-S25. DOI: 10.1053/j.seminoncol.2013.12.002

[44] Mielke J, Jilma B, Koenig F, Jones B. Clinical trials for authorized biosimilars in the European Union: A systematic review. British Journal of Clinical Pharmacology. 2016;**82**(6):1444-1457. DOI: 10.1111/bcp.13076

[45] Jurczak W, Vulto AG, Amersdorffer J, Kim WS, Coiffier B. Research on Biosimilars: Pivotal trials and principles. The Lancet Haematology. 2017;**4**(9):e409-ee10. DOI: 10.1016/S2352-3026(17)30152-7

[46] Schneider CK. Biosimilars in rheumatology: The wind of change. Annals of the Rheumatic Diseases. 2013;**72**(3):315-318. DOI: 10.1136/annrheumdis-2012-202941

[47] Schiestl M, Stangler T, Torella C, Cepeljnik T, Toll H, Grau R. Acceptable changes in quality attributes of glycosylated biopharmaceuticals. Nature Biotechnology. 2011;**29**(4):310-312. DOI: 10.1038/nbt.1839

[48] Tesser JR, Furst DE, Jacobs I. Biosimilars and the extrapolation of indications for inflammatory conditions. Biologics: Targets and Therapy. 2017;**11**:5-11. DOI: 10.2147/BTT.S124476

[49] Weise M, Kurki P, Wolff-Holz E, Bielsky MC, Schneider CK. Biosimilars: The science of extrapolation. Blood. 2014;**124**(22):3191-3196. DOI: 10.1182/blood-2014-06-583617

[50] Lim SH, Beers SA, French RR, Johnson PW, Glennie MJ, Cragg MS. Anti-CD20 monoclonal antibodies: Historical and future perspectives. Haematologica. 2010;**95**(1):135-143. DOI: 10.3324/haematol.2008.001628